How to be "*Hot*" at Sixty

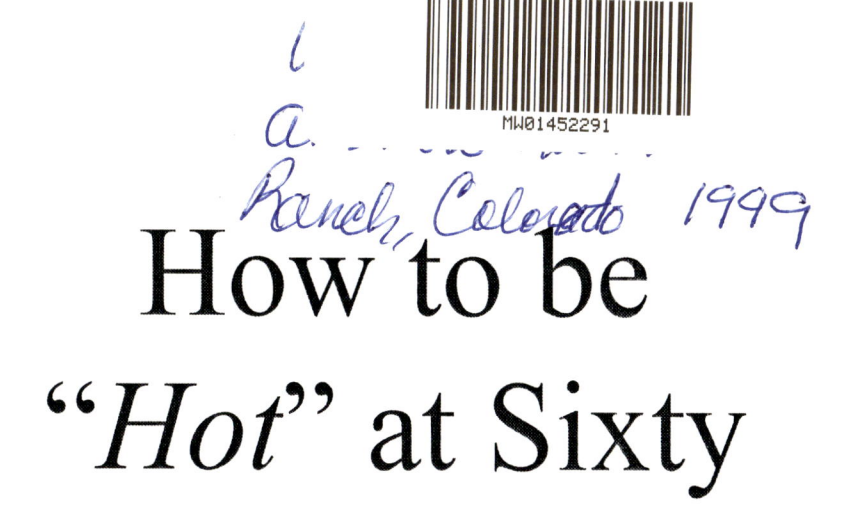

Effie A. Velardo

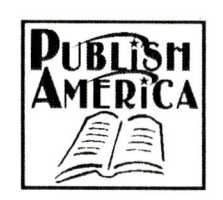

PublishAmerica
Baltimore

© 2003 by Effie A. Velardo.
All rights reserved. No part of this book may be reproduced, stored in a retrieval system, or transmitted in any form or by any means without the prior written permission of the publishers, except by a reviewer who may quote brief passages in a review to be printed in a newspaper, magazine, or journal.

First printing

ISBN: 1-59286-686-7
PUBLISHED BY PUBLISHAMERICA, LLLP
www.publishamerica.com
Baltimore

Printed in the United States of America

Dedication:

As of this writing I am sixty-four years old. My life has been very full and exciting. Although it is far from over, I have had more than my share of tragedies, but also fantastic and wonderful experience's. I have a lot to be thankful for. I also have a lot to take up with God, when I see, him or her. All in all it's been a trip, and when I go, (although I am not in any hurry), I will have no regrets and will leave behind all the things of which I am proudest.

I have tried every day to bring laughter and joy to someone. That I leave behind, seven wonderful children, three sons, Tod, Duncan & Jeremy. They are all very different from one another, but they are all highly intelligent, artistic and handsome. What I love the most about my boys is that they all aspire to their dreams and their ethics, rather than give in to the financial greed of corporate America. To my two absolutely beautiful daughters, Christy and Kelly, (who have most of the children.) Both of these wonderful women are bringing up their children as single parents and managing to balance, work, parenting, fun and responsibility in a way I envy. To my six exceptional grandchildren, Brittany, Zack, & Morgan, Kelly's children and Colby & Cameron, Christy's children, and Josh my youngest grandson, Duncan's son. And finally Alex who in June will become my step grandson. I know all grandparents think that their grandchildren are exceptional, but these kids really are. They are all very artistic, musical, honor roll students and top athletes, I couldn't be prouder.

To all of them I dedicate this book.

To my very wonderful daughter in law Debbie, and my youngest sons life partner, Keith. To my many friends, some who have stood by me for over fifty years, They listen to my babblings and give me strength.

These wonderful people make me look good just by their presence.

Lastly I want to dedicate this book to my Jimmy, the man who puts up with me day to day. He is the soul mate it took me sixty years to find. He is my patient and stable, other half. He builds my confidence and gives me the spark to go on, he diffuses me when I am ready to ignite. He loves me unconditionally. I love you all.

Together you are my life.

How to be Hot at Sixty:

This book is not about my personal life, however in order for you to understand that I am just like you, or perhaps even more disadvantaged, I need to tell you a little about my background.

I have always called the women from my generation, and my mother's generation, "The forgotten women". Why? Because we were really the last generation of women, before the current women's movements in the last twenty or so years.

We came before, "Women's Lib", Equal Rights, and all of the other movements that have sprung up, supposedly to make our lives better and equal.

Ha!! I'm here to tell you it did not work!

It's like the blacks, we are a little better off, but we are far from equal. Few women still, make the same money as men, few work fulltime while their husbands run the home; few have decent retirements or even a good social security.

When the law gets involved, most of the time we loose. For instance now we pay child support, and alimony, but we still do most of the child rearing. My favorite saying during most of the women's lib movements used to be, "if you need a law to get what you want from a man, then you ain't much of a woman." Now that saying sort of intimates that I believe in using feminine wiles to get what I want! Well, I do, but I don't compromise myself in any way while I am doing it! I don't use sexual favors, to climb my way to the top, or to get my own way. The sexuality is there, however, it's an unseen, understood factor. It is the difference between men and women, Vive ala difference!! From Sampson and Delilah, to present day, we have to be aware, that if a woman uses her femininity, even in a subtle way, she can surely get her way with a man. There is a reason men and women are different, we were given our femininity, because men were given brute strength, and we should use that to our advantage.

The law can dictate, that a company has to hire a woman to fill a quota or to be able to get federal funding on a job, the same way they have to hire other minorities. The federal government can use whatever force at its disposal to falsely create equality; but that won't make them like, respect or treat you any better. That's up to you, you can work on a man's job and have them eating out of your hand. If it's to be a positive experience you need more than a law. I think in the past twenty years we have come to realize that.

The intelligent woman will learn to stick up for herself, to be heard, to be pleasant and fair, but to insist on her rights as a person. She must be as strong as is necessary to accomplish her goals, without losing sight of her femininity. Not that I am against any of these movements. I guess in a democracy, it was the only way they could force the issue, or try to. (After all the government and most everything else is ruled by men.) I just don't think they accomplish what they are supposed to. Twenty years later, women are still getting abused by their husbands and bosses every day.

Many women today are still staying in abusive relationships for the security, they believe they have, and for the children. Far less than they used to but still way too many.

I personally know two girls in their thirties who were hired to work on the "Big Dig" in Boston a few years ago, to fill the quota. They were thrilled because the money was indecent, but they don't have a real job. They are making fantastic money as pipe fitters, but they know nothing about "pipe fitting". When they walk around the site, the guys whistle and call out "compliments" etc. occasionally one of the men in charge reprimand them for it but most times not. The girls don't want to complain the paycheck is too good. Is this a gain for equality? There is equality in divorce now, they divide our house down the middle no matter who has the kids, the wife pays child support if she makes as much, I think we lost that battle. We can still work at the same job as a guy and not get paid as much. We are still a long way from becoming president or vice president. We have gained a little in becoming Mayors, governors, or in the house and senate. But look what happened to Jane Swift when she had twins after becoming governor. She was not re-elected and they did not expect her to take any time out to be a mother or to bring her children to her job. Nothing she could do was right.

We are allowed to work outside the home, as long as we can manage to also raise the kids well and run the house. Usually without the help of "you know who", and if he doesn't get enough sex !! Mercy he will divorce you besides. That cute little secretary is always willing to give him that!!

In a lot of ways we are more discriminated against than blacks or other minorities. They can at least go to court and file discrimination charges. When did a woman win a discrimination case in court? That and age discrimination is almost impossible to win.

Well, I am one of those forgotten women, and if you are reading this you can probably relate! We were thought of in our day as merely wives and mothers. Housewives we were called, "Leave it to Beaver Moms". After I had my seventh child I called myself, "An engineer in charge of production" We raised the children, including the boys, and made decent people out of them, because we were always there. We didn't go to work every day. We took the kids to school and picked them up. We worked at the PTA, we ran bake sales, and bazaars, and were brownie moms and Cub Scout leaders.

We taught our girls to set the table properly, and to dance, and sew. We taught our boys to build, and play ball, and to be tough. Certain things were man's work and certain things were women's work. We didn't know any better, that's the way it was for generation after generation. We ran the house, did the budget, (with the money he gave us), took care of the clothing, taxied everyone everywhere, took the kids to the dentist, the doctor, for every lesson that their was from music to horse back riding to tennis. That was what we were good for, nothing else. We did not dare to dream of becoming doctors, or lawyers if we even imagined such a thing we were insane, ungrateful. An ungrateful bitch of a woman that ought to be beat!

We were expected to raise perfect children, keep an immaculate home, always be dressed impeccably, and always ready for your husband. You strove to be a gourmet cook, a financial wizard, a seamstress, teacher, nurse and minister. You were not only responsible for how your children looked, but how they behaved and what they became. If you liked sex you were a whore, if you didn't you were a cold bitch, who's husband had every right to seek his fulfillment elsewhere. You certainly did not have the brains or the time to get involved in business or politics.

My sisters and I were extremely bright, despite our badly dysfunctional family life. I had a grade average of 98.6 in school. I went twelve years to parochial school, including high school. The girls were only allowed to take business courses. I was exceptional in math, biology and Latin, but I could not pursue a course of study in any career that would use these subjects. I could take them as individual courses, but had to take all the secretarial courses.

As a sign of rebellion I got straight A's in math, biology and Latin. I flunked out of shorthand and typing because I did not enjoy it. My teachers were in tears they could not understand me. They made exceptions to the rules, and made me take first year shorthand, and typing two years in a row and gave me my credits both years just because they wanted me to have those skills. The typing did come in handy but the shorthand I soon forgot and never used. Instead I became a bookkeeper for a while and used my math skills.

In those days a woman was not supposed to think about a career, if she did becoming a teacher or a nurse was a respectable profession. Most women were encouraged to dream only of marrying a successful man. College was out of the question for me, so that became my dream too.

My problem was, I was so plain I had no boyfriends, so when a man came along that wanted to marry me, even though he was not particularly attractive and I didn't love him, I married him.

My mother before me was at an even greater disadvantage. She was more than extremely bright, she was a genius. She used to amuse us kids with tales of her traveling on the train with her father in 1921, when she was only three years old. She could recite all the counties in the state of Maine, travelers would give her pennies to do it. She started school at age 5, skipped two grades and graduated from High school at age 16, valedictorian in a class of several hundred in 1934. In her graduation picture she is at least a head shorter than anyone else in her class. For her efforts, she received a one year scholarship, to Salem Commercial school. A secretarial school of course, but my mother was pleased to be able to continue her studies. At the end of the first year, when she wanted to continue, her father said no, education was a waste of time for a girl. Time to stop this foolishness and get married, you silly girl, make a proper home. Enough nonsense! Bold, rebel.

She did get married, within the year to my father. A tall handsome, rouge of a man! He had a fantastic sense of humor. Great personality and a genius in his own right. During his later life he invented many wonderful things, he had an unusual mechanical mind. He was the Errol Flynn of his day, he loved to drink and flirt, he adored my mother but that did not stop his roving eye. He worked for General Electric and I have several awards for $5.00 bonuses he was given for inventions that belonged to the company for which he worked.

My parents tried to have a baby right away, but it was not to be. My mother went to several doctors in an effort to try to find out why. When she finally did get pregnant, two years later it was a standing joke, did I belong to my father or the doctor.

When I arrived, it settled that argument because I was the picture of my father, and he adored me.

I came into the world on December 28th 1938, in the midst of a terrible snowstorm! A premonition of things to come? That storm still stirs within me. For a couple of years my parents were very happy. I was very loved and very spoiled. Three years after me, along came my baby sister. She was my Christmas present, born on December 24th 1941. By now we were into the Second World War. My father did not get into the service, G.E. was making too much for the war effort, but a lot of my cousins and uncles did. My grandfather and uncle worked at the shipyard building submarines.

We were too little to be aware of the war, but blackouts were common. And I remember standing in line for certain items, and adding yellow to white margarine, and stomping on our tin cans and saving them etc.

I loved my baby sister, but my mother made me jealous of her, because she constantly complimented her and insulted me. She favored her greatly, as she looked like her. Every day when she brushed our hair she would remark about how thin and miserable mine was and how thick and lustrous hers was. My sister had a head full of auburn curls that were gorgeous. My mother's comments affected me so much that one day, I cut off all my sisters curls. By this time my hair had grown just enough to have two tiny braids, one on each side of my head. My punishment, was my mother cut off my braids. I was devastated, but I had learned my lesson. No matter how jealous I was I took good care of my sister from then on. I was still my fathers, favorite although he did not show it the way my mother did.

Even at my tender age, I learned to avoid my mother's temper. I remember one Christmas, I got two beautiful dolls. One looked like a princess and the other was a soldier doll. I loved them both, but I was still a baby really, five years old. My mother had apparently told me several times to pick up my toys, when I was done playing them. I did not and the next thing I knew she had picked up the boy doll by the ankles and smashed his head into a million pieces. I cried and cried but it did no good, I learned. I also soon learned to stay out of my mothers way when she was in one of these rages.

Our life was not bad in those days, because as strict and mean as my mother could be, my dad was fun and funny. He had a fantastic love for animals and a real knack for training even wild ones. I remember for a time that we had mallard ducks in our bathtub. We always had dogs and kittens. My dad went hunting with my grandfather one day and brought home a live, horned owl on a lease. The owl was a full sized adult that had been crippled and my father kept him and nursed him back to health. He kept it in a cage down cellar until it was well. Then one night the bird broke right thru the cage and the cellar window to freedom. My dad could train a dog to do anything, we had one that could only understand French, and another that would only take food out of your left hand.

One night, during a blackout, we heard my mother crying. My father had not come home from work. Apparently my father had been having an affair or two. My parents divorced. We moved out of our cute little home and in with my aunt in Kittery Maine, in a little naval village outside of the Navy yard. My mother did not live with us, she had an apartment in Dover, she went to work in a factory for the war effort. My father lived in Lynn, Mass. near G.E. My aunt Polly was my mother's younger sister. She was very nice but she already had three boys of her own, and the house was tiny. We did love my cousins and enjoyed having them to play with. We lived with them for a couple of years. My uncle worked at the navy yard with my grandfather. They would often take us to the navy yard to see them launch a new submarine. Our life was okay, my sister missed my mother terribly and she cried and hung on me all the time. I was like her surrogate mother even though I was only six. She was always crying, I was unhappy too, but I knew I had to be strong for her. My aunt was good to us, but it was hard for her trying to support seven people in that little house with a war going on and all that went with it. The shortages, and the rationing. My father helped her as much as he could but probably not enough. In those days the courts didn't necessarily get involved like they do now. We were all little so it did not influence us that much personally. We enjoyed playing bombers in the old apple tree in the back yard, we would sit up in the branches and drop red salmon bricks down to the ground. One day I had one drop on my head. Believe it or not no damage, didn't even split my head. There was a large wooded area at the end of our street and we played a lot there. We would collect snakes and put them in people's mailboxes or put them in glass milk bottles. Or we would pretend we were stalking German prisoners who had escaped from the military prison at the Navy yard.

My aunt naturally favored her own children, and I was always getting into trouble with my oldest cousin who loved setting me up and then tattling to my aunt so I would get a spanking. Sometimes we would get all the neighborhood kids together and have a C.Y.O. show at the end of the street. I loved to sing and was always the star of the show.

My dad still worked at G.E. in Lynn, but he would ride his motorcycle down on the weekends and take my sister and I back to Lynn on the train to his apartment. We lived for those weekends, he lived right on the beach in a big apartment building. He bought us all kinds of great toys and kept them at his place for us to use on the weekends. We even had a toy iron that really heated up. When it was nice we would play on the beach, run in the sand and water. My dad would take movies of us. I remember he had a friend who lived upstairs who played the banjo for us, we loved it.

My mother was working in a plant in Dover making something for the navy, she was the original "Rosie the Riveter". She probably liked it much better than being a housewife. Unfortunately, her becoming pregnant shortened her freedom by a man much older than herself. In those days if that happened you got married. There was no other choice. My dad always used to tell me that if it didn't happen he and my mother would have gotten back together. Who knows. The man was twenty years older than my mother. A fifty year old, Irish bachelor. He and my mother got married and moved into a home he bought her in Newburyport, Mass. My sister and I went there to live. Very soon after my mother had a new baby, another sister Eleanor. My stepfather Tom, absolutely adored the baby, you would have thought she was the only one ever born. We adored her too, and were happy to be back with my mother. She was no better homemaker than before however, and I took care of the baby most of the time. By now I was about seven or eight. My stepfather was very good to us, he bought Flo and I both new dolls. He never spanked us or yelled at us. We were a little afraid of him though because he was an old man and a stranger. My mother did her duties, she was a great cook, she kept a neat home, she was a fantastic seamstress, and even took in sewing for other people. Her heart just wasn't in it. I can still see her stretching those dam curtains on the curtain stretchers out in the yard. As time went on, she became very restless. She needed something to stimulate her mind, she loved socializing. She was always in the back or side yard talking over the fence with the neighbors. She visited back and forth with them. She used to stand at our front gate leaning on her elbows talking with anyone who walked by. She was starved for outside knowledge. Everyone knew her, she socialized with the merchants up town. She did work for some of them. To earn extra merchandise. We never had a car, not too many people did. My grandparents did, we considered them rich. But we never did, so we were confined to things within walking distance. Down town was only about three blocks so we often walked there. Our school was about five blocks so we walked that four times a day, because we came home for lunch. My mother walked to town a lot. She had a group of old friends she had since high school that she kept in touch with. They would get together a couple of times a month. They called it a sewing club, but they mostly talked and munched. It was a social club. My mother loved clothes, especially hats, even though she had few places to wear them. She could not afford them, on the allowance my father gave her so she sewed for a milliner up town and in turn she would give her deals on hats. My stepfather was a good man, but he didn't have a clue at his advanced age what it took to support a family. He gave my mother $40.00 a week to support the whole family. Food, clothes, heat, utilities and any extras all came out of that. The milk bill, gifts etc. My mother would never tell him it was impossible to do. To her that would have been failure. So instead, she tried to make it up with her sewing money. She got further and further behind. My stepfather was very jealous, because she was so attractive and he was so much older. So he never took her anywhere. He was so jealous of my father coming to visit us that he struck a deal with him. He convinced him it was too hard on us seeing him and then him leaving and that it would be more stable for us not to see him. He told him if he would stop coming and move away he would not have to ever pay child support again. My father believing it to be true, and wanting to move on with his own life, moved to California. We kept in touch by mail, but didn't see him for many years. My stepfather continued to favor his daughter, but we didn't care. He treated us well and left us alone. Three years after his first child my mother had another baby this time a boy. She was thrilled her first son, my stepfather strangely still favored his daughter, and was very strict with his son. The baby was named after him, Tommy. We were thrilled to have a baby brother, I took care of him all the time. He was adorable with golden curls, my mother adored him but still left most of the mothering to me. By now I was about eleven, and was quite the bossy little mother.

My mother favored my brother and my sister Flo, My stepfather favored Eleanor his daughter. I had been my dad's favorite but he was gone. I had no one to love me but the babies, so I really made over them and they loved me. They gave me the affection I so craved. My mother barked orders at me all the time. If I was not in school I was baby-sitting even if she was there. I watched them, dressed them, fed them and disciplined them. I got very little for my efforts. I never ever had a new dress, one pair of shoes, for school only if I needed it and my mother made my coats or they were hand me down from cousins. As a result, when I was anywhere but home, I was very shy and intimidated. In school I was a perfect student but very self-conscious and not at all social. The kids I went to school with were all wealthy. The children of doctors, lawyers, dentists, undertakers etc. one's father was a judge. They all had plenty of free time to socialize and play. My only close friends were girls from the neighborhood who were as much social outcasts as I was. They went to public school, I went to private financed by Tom's sister who had a lot of money and thought we should go to Christian school. We hung around together all our lives and are still friends today. My mother continued as we grew to praise my sister in front of me. She told her how pretty she was, and lived through her. I was just the maid. If I complained about doing something she wanted me to do, she would either hit me with the belt or threaten to commit suicide.

I knew even then, that she was frustrated at not being able to live her life the way she wanted to. I understood, because I was the same way. Luckily however I did not take after her, I was my father's daughter, I had his sense of humor and ability to land on my feet no matter what. I was very different from my mother, I always had a knack for making the best of my situation or finding a way to get what I wanted even when I was young. At home I was always joking around, and I was basically happy even in my miserable skin. My stepfather called me "Gracie" for Gracie Allen a comedian of the time.

He thought I was very funny. I had my fantasies, I brought them to life in drawing and designing. I was always sitting at the dining room table drawing. I drew a comic strip in which we were the main characters, but we had a wonderful life in my strip.

I collected paper dolls of all the movie stars, you could buy a paper doll book at the corner store in those days for a few pennies. Or they would come free in the weekly or Sunday paper. I had a big box of all the movie stars from the 30's and 40's. Rita Hayworth, Hedy Lamar, Deanna Durbin, Lana Turner and Shirley Temple. Sonia Henie and Barbara Stanwick, I was fascinated by them. I would cut out the dolls and design wonderful dresses and gown for them. That I got from my mother, she loved to design clothes. Another time, another place either of us would have been a great designer.

My mother became more and more unhappy, she wanted so much to go out and socialize but she would not communicate this to my stepfather. His idea of a social life was, on Friday night at the end of the week, he would bring home a bottle of liquor. After the kids were in bed. He and my mother would sit on the living room couch talking and drinking, until they got drunk. Then he would screw her all night. I would lie up in my bed and listen to them. They would start off laughing and talking and then you would hear the noises of their love making. One time I crept downstairs and saw my mother laying naked on the couch. I was disgusted, even though I really didn't know what they were doing. All I knew was my mother did not look like she was having fun. Years later I found out, it was just another frustrating experience for her. She told her friend, he would get her all riled up and then come off himself and leave her frustrated. My mother was a very sexual person, I am sure this was very upsetting to her and contributed to her depression and mental state later.

My mother began going down hill more and more. Financially her debts were getting out of hand and she feared my stepfather finding out. Physically she suffered from and over or under active thyroid, whichever one makes you get fat. She took diet pills, then other pills to calm her down. She became an alcoholic as a result of their Friday night drinking binges. Her father had been an alcoholic and she should never have been subjected to that amount of alcohol. My stepfather didn't realize, it didn't effect him the same way. Her mental capacity diminished, she cried she threatened suicide more and more. Only to us though not to him.

My stepfather never gave her any more money, even when things went up. She could not keep up with the sewing. She continued to make herself nice clothes even though she had no place to go. She just liked having them. She would get dressed up just to work around the house or to go up town.

My sisters and I and our girl friends tried to live a normal life. In the summer we would put blankets on the front lawn and play dolls. We always pretended to be a movie star, I was Dale Evans married to Roy Rogers. My sister Flo liked to be Linda Darnell married to Victor Mature. We lived in our fantasy world, it made our every day life bearable. As we got older we went to the movies a lot, we loved the old musicals. We would come out singing and tap dancing. Now we became, Doris Day, Ginger Rogers, Kathryn Grayson, we dreamed about Fred Astaire, Donald O'Connor, Johnny Ray, Gorden MacRae, Edmund Purdom and Mario Lanza.

Our real life was so far removed from this life. During all the time I was growing up I never had a new dress or coat from a store. When I was thirteen I started selling blueberries for the lady next door. I made a nickel a box with my earnings that summer I was able to buy a storm coat for school that year. I was so proud of that coat, I can't tell you. The year I went to High school my mother made me a couple of swing skirts, and blouses. Middy blouses were in, and saddle shoes and bobbie sox and ponytails.

In my freshman year I was miraculously invited to the prom, by a boy I liked. It was unbelievable for me, and for once my mother was happy for me and made me a gown. It was bright red! With black netting around the shoulders, but at the time I thought it was beautiful. I think that one time she was proud of me.

When we were young, every Easter she would make us all Easter outfits. They would all match, My mother and us three girls. Tommy she would dress in a little man's outfit including a little topcoat and soft hat. When we were little it was cute, but she continued the practice into our teens and then it was embarrassing. We hated it, but she loved it. Of course people would compliment her on it and she loved that and would try to outdo herself the following year.

My mother continued to drink, it got worse and worse. Their Friday nights continued. I think she drank, to keep up with him, and to forget and to numb herself for the lovemaking sessions. Their social nights began to get ugly, they would start talking in a normal tone, but it would swiftly turn into a nasty shouting match, the drunker they got the louder they became. Then it would turn into a fight, sometimes even to blows. My mother was getting fed up with never going out and giving into him, but unless she was drunk she did not have the courage to tell him. As I got older she confided in me as though I was her best buddy. She talked to me about their sex life and how unsatisfying it was for her. In those days however like everything else the woman was just supposed to be there to satisfy her man. A woman was not supposed to enjoy sex. I listened but I had no idea what she was talking about. I didn't find out about the sex act till I was seventeen years old. One of the advantages of going to a parochial school. It meant little to me, but I tried to be sympathetic. I knew she was becoming more and more stressed and I knew she was very unhappy but I had no idea how to help her. Then she began drinking when it wasn't Friday night. The only excuse she had for leaving the house by herself was to go grocery shopping. It became a ritual for us. Every Friday night we would go uptown to go grocery shopping.

Before we would go to the store she would take me to a bar in a hotel. She would have a few drinks at the bar, and socialize. while I had a coke and waited for her. Then we would hurry to the grocery store and hurry home.

My stepfather never got suspicious for some reason. Then they would start drinking and they would fight so bad, I would have to get up and yell at them. Liquor was expensive, she got herself in so deep financially, that she decided to go to work. My stepfather was not happy about her decision but I think by this time he could see she needed a diversion. She began working a night shift at the Hytron Company. Her alcoholism continued, she was still taking the diet pills, the Thyroid pills and Benzadrine. She would go to work every afternoon at 3:00 and home about eleven. My stepfather didn't like it, she was becoming more independent, and the booze gave her courage. She told me she wanted to leave him, but she didn't tell him. She wanted to take my sister Flo and me, but leave the two youngest, his two. I told her I could not leave the babies with him . Again she threatened to commit suicide, she had a bottle of some kind of poison and she would pull it out and threaten to drink it and I would give in to her. This time though I refused to give in. I told her I would not go with her. Then one night she just didn't come home from work.

My step dad, woke me about three in the morning. Your mother didn't come home, I'm worried sick. I got a sick feeling in my stomach. I got up and sat with him, all night. By morning I knew she had gone, I started telling my stepfather, what she had been going through, and how she had threatened to leave. The next day he called her family, her parents came we called the police etc. but she was never found, not a trace.

At first it was very hard, I was sixteen, my younger siblings ranged from thirteen to five. Now I really had to come right home from school and take care of the babies. My thirteen year old sister and me did everything, we cleaned the house, took care of the kids, cooked etc. My father came on from California to take my sister and I back, but we wouldn't go. I would have loved to, but I could not leave the two little ones. It was devastating enough for them to have no mother, if my sister and I left them, heaven knows what would have happened to them. We went to court with my stepfather to tell the judge we wanted to stay with him. My father was devastated but I tried to explain to him. My High school teacher caught me crying in class more than once.

We survived though, through my high school life, I could not go anywhere with the other kids after school, I could not participate in any after school activities, every day right home to take care of the kids. I became more and more of an outsider, more with drawn, more shy and intimidated. The other kids I went to Parochial school with were all very well to do, sons and daughters of local doctors, dentists, undertakers, they all had money and clothes. They went to parties, and skiing, and were involved in sports or cheerleading. My only outside activity at school was the band.

My sister and I were both in the band and we did get to go to different places to be in parades. The only reason my sister and I could even afford to go to the private school was my stepfathers sister had always paid our tuition.

He had two sisters that were fairly well to do. Of course they had no idea what went on in our home between their brother and my mother. They were shocked when she left.

I dreamed about dating, and boys , but no one ever asked me out. My younger sister was very popular, she was very pretty and she was always being asked out. The few men I met including my first husband were boys she brought home. I had to keep a sharp eye on her, because she was only thirteen and she would make out with anybody, I'm sure she was trying to make up for the lack of love she got at home.

I made up my mind that neither of us was going to get pregnant, or do anything to make people think any less of us than they already did. Most people who heard about my mother, looked down their noses at us, and expected the worst. I was totally dedicated to staying a virgin till I got married, if that ever happened, and to keeping my sister the same. My little sister was nine and my brother was five. I was their mother, I cooked, cleaned did their laundry and tried to keep my stepfather going. He was retired from his company but he worked as a bartender at the nearby D.A.V. club.

As young as I was I was always very strong willed. I knew what I wanted out of life. The problem, I had no money, and no way to make any. My sister broke up with one guy, who took it very hard. He was about five years older than she was, he had a car. In those days no one had cars, so this made him very attractive, even though he wasn't. He kept hanging around our house, and crying on my shoulder, probably hoping she would come back to him. As we got to know each other, we started going out. It was exciting to me, because I had never gone out before. Going to a drive in movie or having him buy me something to eat was a whole new world. He started coming baby sitting with me. I had never made out with a guy before, so when he started to make out with me, it felt pretty good. I was not particularly attracted to this guy, but it was all I had at the time. By this time I was thoroughly convinced, that I was too ugly to ever get a man. The longer we went out the more involved we got, but I would never go all the way with him, I was not going to get pregnant.

Eventually, he asked me to marry him. I had gone out with him through out my last two years of High school, and when he gave me a diamond in my senior year, I couldn't wait to show it off. All the girls envied me, and for the first time I was the center of attention. I got one of the leads in the senior play, and for the last few months of school, I became fairly popular.

I should have read the signs, and pulled back. I was young and stupid and starry eyed and a year later I married him. I knew I didn't love him, but for the first time I felt that my life was my own.

At first, I had tried to change the course of my life. When I first got out of High school, I moved to Maine, to live with the same aunt that I had been with as a baby. I got a job working in the office of the shoe shop in her town. I tried to get away from my fiancée, because I knew I didn't love him. I was smart enough to know I had to try for an alternative. I even met a couple of boys down there, through my male cousins. My fiancée came down every weekend to see me and take me out. I tried one time to break up with him, and he cried. I felt trapped, and at my young age didn't know how to handle it. I moved back home.

We moved into an apartment only a couple of blocks away from my home. I could still help to look after the kids and my father. My younger sister was now sixteen and she more or less took over, the other kids were eight and fourteen and they had fallen into a routine of looking after themselves pretty well.

At first it was great being married, I had my own job, my own apartment, I could buy my own clothes, buy furniture and decorated my own place. Things I had never had or never done in my life! It was like playing house. I never once thought about it as a lifetime commitment, even though I had resolved to never put my kids through what I had gone through. It had been a convenient way to get out of a situation. I did not love my husband, but we were good friends, he was very good to me, he let me have control of the finances and to buy anything I thought we could afford.

I bought lots of clothes, and hats and shoes. I worked in an office doing payroll, and I was the best-dressed woman in the office. Men began to look at me, and come on to me. It was a whole new thing to me, but I was not ever going to be disloyal to my husband. I had a very strong moral background, from the Catholic school. You would go to hell if you ever cheated on your husband, even in your mind ! My worst fears were that I would end up like my mother that was always in the back of my mind. I got my love of clothes, and hats, and independence from her, my mathematical mind. I had my fathers, good sense, and how to deal with people, his great sense of humor, and I guess his good looks . Once I was no longer around the people who intimidated me I began to shine. I was a survivor, I could take any amount of abuse, as long as it got me what I wanted in the end. I think that's the way I looked at my marriage. A means to an end. All it cost me was being a good wife to my husband, and I could have everything else I wanted.

I had been doing bookkeeping from the time I was sixteen, I was always good in figures, so I had a good job. I was popular at work, the men thought I was sexy and the women loved my sense of humor. I would go around and get everyone's lunch orders and go out to get them.

My life was comfortable, I wanted a baby right away but I hated having sex with my husband. When we first got married it took almost two weeks before we actually, consummated our marriage. When we did have sex it had to be just straight sex, nothing kinky, no oral stuff. I was certainly sexual enough, if I thought of someone else, I could always have an orgasm. I just didn't like him that well. Everything else in the marriage was fine. In those days, most women said they hated sex, so I guess I just thought it was normal. The women I worked with, considered it their wifely duties, no one talked about it like they loved it.

In the second year of our marriage, we still had not gotten pregnant. I thought there must be something wrong with one of us. My husband was up for the draft, as all young men were in those days. If we got pregnant he could be deferred, but we hadn't. He did not want to get drafted into the Army. If he had to go in the service, he wanted it to be the Air Force. So when the second year came and still no baby, he enlisted in the Air Force.

The day he signed on the dotted line, I missed my period. By the time he went to boot camp, I was six months along. It was too late, he was in for four years. I wasn't worried though, I could go to the service doctors for my prenatal care at the Navy base, where my uncle and grandfather still worked.

I learned to drive the car, so I could use it while he was away. It was kind of great having him gone! I moved back in with my step dad who was thrilled to have me.

When my husband got out of boot camp, I was eight months along. His first tour of duty was Hamilton field, in Novato California. Novato is just over the Golden Gate in San Francisco. That sounded so exciting to me. My husband wanted me to stay home and have the baby there, and join him later. I had already gone through most of the pregnancy alone, he was going to be there for the baby's birth. I insisted on going with him.

We turned in the plane ticket the Air Force had given him, and used the money for gas and the trip out. My father lived in Long Beach, it was the other end of California, but it was the same state. I had no idea how long California was! I called him and told him I was coming out to stay till I had my baby! He was delighted, (I'm not sure his new wife was). We drove cross-country, it was the first time I had ever been further than Boston. It was wonderful seeing the country, even though we went Highways and were on a time limit. We had to be there in four days. For kids like us it was the adventure of a lifetime! We got to Long Beach, my husband met my dad, dropped me off and continued to his assigned base.

It was great over that month getting to know my dad again. He was the same as I remembered him. Fun, humorous, smart, determined, and stubborn. He had definite ideas about everything. His wife was sweet, but she was definitely dominated by him. I would give him an argument about everything and she would get a great kick out of it. She could not get over how alike we were.

Dad still called me "schmickelpuss" a name he had called me as a baby. We had a lot of the same habits, even though we had not lived together since I was six. We both covered our baked beans with molasses, for instance. We walked alike, had a lot of the same mannerisms. We would both hug ourselves and rock when we were sitting talking to someone. Finally the night came when the baby was born. My dad raced me to the Hospital, and stayed with me through a long labor, and the baby's birth. I had gotten a really great doctor when I got to Long Beach and he was wonderful through out the birth process. He sat up a three-way mirror so I could see everything. It was the most wonderful experience of my life, even though I was terribly sick to my stomach through the entire thing. It was a gorgeous girl, just what I wanted, I had her name picked out for a year. Kelly jean. My husband was in the same State but 800 miles away. We called him and he came down the next day. Everyone was delighted, the baby was gorgeous.

Three days later, we took off by car, for San Francisco. We had a new baby, no money, and no place to live, and we had to go 800 miles.

My dad had given us $60.00 which in those days, was a months rent in most places. My husband was only an Airman third class, which was basically no rank. We had to leave all our furniture etc stored on the East coast. We were basically starting off with nothing.

The trip up the State was terribly, It was June, very hot. Our car had no air conditioning, by the time we got to Fresno, the baby had a terrible heat rash and was crying constantly! The car overheated. We pulled over into a park, I stripped off all her clothes and let the air blow on her. By dark we got into San Rafael, the town next to the Air Base. We paid a months rent on a motel room, that had a combination, stove refrigerator, as well as a chair and a bed. That was our home for a month. Right off a busy highway, with no sidewalks. I thought I would go nuts, but I loved having the baby and tried to just enjoy her.

At the end of the first month, when he got his meager paycheck, we moved. This time to a motel type unit, but it had a combination kitchen, living room and separate bedroom, and it was in town. It was also fully furnished. So we began our new life there. He would go to the Air Base every day. I would clean the place, take the baby for a walk and get social with the neighbors. I used cloth diapers and I had to walk to a laundromat with the baby's laundry every day.

We wound up living in California, for the entire four years, my husband was in the Air Force. It was not a fun time in general, but we did have a lot of fun times mixed with the misery. It was a great time of learning, we matured a lot. I had always been forced into a role that was way beyond my years, but now I had to make a life for myself. We were a couple of kids, 3000 miles from home and family and friends. We had no one to depend on but each other.

My husband made a very small salary, because he was a draftsman, he got to know a lot of officers who helped him out. He would make signs for the Commissary for instance and the guy would give him some steaks. He had a couple of single friends who would come by and give us a hand once in a while. I got pregnant immediately again, and within nine months had a second little girl. Kelly had been born in June, and the following April Paula was born. Paula was born perfectly healthy, but she weighed only five pounds. She was a preemie. Air Force hospitals are not the cleanest there are.

She caught pneumonia, as did three other babies in the nursery. They all weighed more than she did. Paula passed away after struggling to breathe for three days. I stood at that incubator and willed her to breathe, but she didn't make it. I was devastated, as was my husband and our friends. I was twenty one years old, I had a baby at home, and now I had to bury one. We had no money and no one to tell us how to go about it. Someone directed us to a Church cemetery that had a special baby lot. We made arrangements and they let us bury her there for nothing. We took the little white casket to the cemetery in a station wagon. A few prayers were said and that was that. I left my precious baby there.

A month later, I told my husband I could not take it any more. I had to go home. I was terribly homesick. I took Kelly, who was almost a year old. I filled a knapsack with baby food and dry milk. I took the money we were supposed to pay the rent with that month, and got on a Grey Hound bus for Boston.

My baby and I had climbed on the bus in San Francisco, after we bought our ticket, we had $10.00 for the trip. The look on my husband's face when he put us on, was one of, he would never see us again! We headed home.

The baby was great on the trip. She was just learning to walk, and toddled everywhere. Everyone on the bus loved her, and they would treat us to meals when we stopped. The bus trip was a grand adventure, unlike a car trip, the bus goes through all the big cities. I enjoyed seeing all the new places. We had to sleep on the bus, we met lots of nice people. Old ladies and service men were especially kind. They would fall in love with the baby and buy us dinner. It took four days, and we were home.

It was great catching up with everybody and showing the baby off. No one had seen her, so we were welcome everywhere, my grandparents, her grandparents. My friends some of whom had babies of their own her age. After we were home a month, however, I realized we had to get back. Her father thought we had abandoned him, and we had to get back to reality. I was over my feeling sorry for myself. I had to go to work in a sandwich shop for a few weeks to earn our airfare back. We flew back to Frisco. My husband was overjoyed to see us. So overjoyed I got pregnant right away again! Then another tragedy, Kelly was fourteen months old and into everything. In my house I had baby proofed everything. We were at a girlfriends for coffee one morning. We were all drinking coffee and chatting. Kelly was toddling around with other babies playing. She came over to me and handed me a bottle she had taken off a windowsill, she had apparently been drinking out of it. It was ant poison, I read the ingredients. Arsenic!! I got up screaming, and immediately picked her up, and took her to the sink. I poured a jar of warm salt water down her throat and made her vomit. Then I called the Air Base, they told me they would have an ambulance at the front gate waiting but they were not allowed to come into town to pick her up. We had to get out to the base and none of us girls had cars. I picked Kelly up and ran the few blocks to downtown with her hoping to find someone to help. I saw a police car in a gas station and flagged him down. He told me the Air Base was out of his jurisdiction, but he could take me to a local hospital. I was in his cruiser by this time. I was upset as I knew the ambulance was already waiting at the gate but we were on our way to the local hospital. Once there, they took their time about getting her checked and finding a doctor etc. I began to cry, I was getting more upset by the minute, the policeman was still there with me. I told him about recently loosing my other baby, and how I could not loose this one. He took pity on me and put us back in the cruiser and we went 100 miles an hour to the Air Base. Sirens blaring, and lights flashing. The ambulance was where it said it would be, they took the baby from me and started immediately pumping her stomach etc. The next twenty four hours were critical. I stayed over night with her. They said she could be paralyzed for life or her organs could be damaged etc. She ran around and raised hell all night she was fine!! The next day a reporter from the San Francisco Examiner came and took her picture and gave her a big new doll. It was on the front page of the paper, with a story praising the officers quick thinking at getting her to the base on time!!

Less than a week after that experience, we were getting ready to go to bed one night. We almost always went to bed by 10:00 - 10:30 at the latest. One night a week we stayed up later to watch some favorite show we had at the time. It happened to be that particular night. We had only one bedroom. The baby was asleep in her crib, across the bedroom from our bed. Actually across the room but at the very foot of our bed. At eleven after our show we went to bed.

We had heard a sound like a backfire about 10:15 - 10:30 but thought nothing of it. We crawled into bed in the dark, so not to disturb the baby. As I started to go to sleep, I put my hand under my pillow, as is my habit. I felt something fuzzy and commented on it to my husband. He felt the fuzzy stuff and put on the light. We picked up my pillow, there was fuzzy stuff like stuffing from the mattress all under my pillow.

I was puzzled as to what it was, but my husband started feeling down the mattress, till he came to a lump. He tore off the sheet and cut the mattress at the bump with a knife. He pulled out a bullet ! Then we looked in the wall, just over my pillow was a bullet hole! We called the police, a sniper had shot a hole in our wall, and it had gone into our mattress. If we had gone to bed on time, it would have gone right through the top of my head, killing my unborn child and me. If it had not hit the mattress it would have hit Kelly in her crib. The sniper was never discovered. We made the papers the next day .

The following year on May 2, I gave birth to my first son. I had never wanted a boy, but after loosing my second daughter, I stopped caring what sex the child was and prayed for the baby to be healthy.

He was gorgeous and perfect. An absolutely beautiful baby, thick curly dark hair, even tempered, good baby. Wonderful personality, never cried, would eat and sleep and play. I could put him out on the lawn in his playpen and he would watch the neighborhood kids play and never fuss. Kelly loved him and he helped amuse her. She had always been a terrible baby, the type who was colicky, and cry every night when you put her to bed. I could never have a baby sitter with her, after one time no one would watch her again. Kip was different he was so good natured he would stay with anybody.

We had been in California two years and had three children, my husband was only an airman third, the bottom of the barrel. Which meant his paycheck was not enough to support a family. In order to make it we had to move in with another young couple or we would have starved.

At Christmas we were given the Welfare basket for being the youngest and neediest airman on the base. Somehow we made it, but it certainly was not easy. Just before Kip was born, I started raising hell, about my baby dying in an Air Force hospital.

I had gone to the chaplain and asked about suing the service, because I found out the survival rate of infants at the air base was far less than those born in town. He told me you can't sue the government, but between that and my husbands connections with officers he worked with, we were all of a sudden given base housing. That was unheard of for an airman third class.

Once we moved on base, things got much easier. We still had no money, but we had our own townhouse, we didn't have to share with anyone else. There were two bedrooms, an up and down stairs and a nice yard for the kids. It was a nice social atmosphere too. There was like four townhouses all connected with one central big yard, both front and back and they were all service wives and kids in the same boat more or less.

We made some good friends that stayed with us to this day. My house became the place for the women to gather for apple pie and coffee each day. Then they would take their babies home for their naps and house clean and later in the day we would get together on the front lawn and discuss the soap operas while the kids played.

Eleven months after Kip was born, I had yet another baby. Another girl, Christy, now I had four children in three years, the oldest only three.

We stayed in California until my husband was discharged, we had been there four years. We drove cross-country with our three surviving babies to start over again. All the furniture and baby stuff we had acquired we had to leave there because we still did not have enough rank or money to ship everything. We did have our furniture from before stored at my fathers, but there was no beds or anything for the babies.

The only thing that bothered me to leave behind, however was my baby. I hated leaving Paula behind in the little baby lot of the cemetery. I had no choice. The four years away had taught us a lot.

We had to depend entirely on each other, and our friends. Our families had been over 3000 miles away. We had become independent and responsible for a couple of kids, I was only twenty four, and the mother of three children. My husband was twenty six and responsible for our care. Luckily he had a job to come back to, the same one he had when he went in the service.

We had no place to live again, and had to buy basics for the kids right away. We somehow managed to borrow $2,000.00 from his employer and we rented a place and bought what we needed. It was ok for a while, but it was not the best neighborhood. We lived there maybe a year and my kids got bugs from kids in the neighborhood. That was it for me ! We were moving!

I called a realtor, and told him I had no money, but I needed a house. Everyone told me I was crazy, you couldn't buy a house with no money down! But, in the end, I did! He found me a beautiful four-bedroom home in a great section of town. I had not wanted to pay over $10,000.00 this one was $13,000.00 but they agreed to finance it and we bought it.

My husband was worried sick because we had never paid over $65.00 a month for a rental, this was going to be $104.00 a month with the taxes and insurance. I made up my mind I would make it, and I did we had that house for twenty seven years.

Again our house became the hub for everything that was going on. I introduced myself to all my neighbors and started inviting them over for coffee klatches, apple pie, coffee and conversation. I introduced all the neighbors to each other, until I moved in a lot of them did not know one another. It was a very compatible neighborhood, for five houses on both sides up the street, they were all catholic and all had three children or more. So it was a great place for my kids to grow up. It was like an extended family, we all shared the same general morals and attitudes and helped out with one another's children.

That is the one thing lacking in the world today, that extended family feeling. As good as my social life and time with my kids was, however, my life with my husband was not. Outside the home, I was this happy social funny person. In the house, I was still intimidated, my husband intimidated me.

He was extremely jealous, and not very social himself. He would have jealous rages, and fly into a temper fit over nothing. He was not a strong man, he was generally very quiet. Apparently the years of being intimidated at school, and having my mother tell me I was unattractive, had cause this basic self consciousness in me. His furious temper when he was jealous, scared me into submission, as a result if we were out at a school function or work party I would not dare be a social butterfly. He did not want me to dance with anyone else, even a good friend.

If he thought I was being too friendly we would have to leave. Other than our social life, he allowed me to control, the money, the house, the children, our purchases and vacations. I personally belonged to him! I think part of it was the basic lack of security that all women felt in those days. We didn't work, which was good for the family unit and the kids., but it kept us bound to our husbands for our security.

Therefore, every woman I know felt, if you get out of line, your husband has the right to throw you out and then what will you do.? That thought alone kept most of us in line. We were dependent on our husbands for everything, our house, our food our clothing, and the children.

The church that we all belonged to, taught us that our body belonged to our husband. I remember getting into a fierce debate with a priest one time about that very issue. I told him, this is my body, not his and I will decide what to do with it. He said no it belongs to your husband! So, when I was out with my husband, I reverted back to the self-conscious person I had been throughout school. We often had parties at our house, especially at Halloween. One such party my husband punched out his first cousin for asking me to dance in our own home. These kind of instances, caused us to be unpopular with our friends as a couple. They all got along great with me during the day, and with the kids functions but when they all joined the country club, or tennis club etc. they did not ask us.

My husband did not particularly want a lot of children. I think he was jealous of the time I put into them as well, but he liked me being "barefoot and pregnant" as they said in those days. He knew the children would keep me at home. Within a year of returning from California we bought the house, the following year we had another baby, a boy Tod.

The kids and I had a good time, everyday when they were little, we would take the big old English carriage that I had, and we would walk downtown. The carriage was huge, and I could fit three kids in the carriage, the older ones would walk, or if they got tired they would ride on the fender of the carriage. We also had the neighbors and their kids over everyday for snacks and conversation and play for the kids.

We had a very big yard, and we bought one of the first above ground pools. My husband built a big deck on it and in the summer the other mothers and I would sit out there and teach the kids to swim and play in the pool.

As the kids got older, they all became involved in the same things at the same time. Brownies, boy scouts, cub scouts, little league, pioneer league and school basketball. The parents all coached or taught. Nearly every night we were at the ballpark.

We volunteered in the P.T.O. which my husband and I were presidents of for over eight years. We volunteered for the ball park snack bar, and the parish counsel, and bingo. During the years, we were presidents of the P.T.O. we planned many bazaars, dinner dances and other activities to raise money for the Parochial school all our children went to . It was a very busy and full life.

As I became more involved in these things, I began to deeply resent my husbands hold over me. I started to revolt, which would always end in a fight. Slowly but surely though I began to pull away from his authority. One of the times we were at a school dance and I danced with a friend and he said we are going home, I said no, you are going home, I am staying. He stayed but didn't speak to anyone all night.

We were not rich by any means, but we had enough to get along on , and to have a vacation every year. Even though none of the mothers worked, we could afford a nice home, two cars, a pool. Our children had all the best, all types of lessons, music, dancing, gymnastics. They had the best clothes and all the latest toys. The children were beautiful, healthy and well rounded. I had lots of friends and was totally involved.

Then tragedy struck again. My five-year-old son, got leukemia! He was so beautiful and healthy looking I could not believe it. Leukemia was a disease I had always dreaded, because when I was a kid a neighbor child had died of it and I always remembered him.

Kip had just gotten over the flu, and he didn't seem to bounce back like his usual self. He had remained listless, and tired. He kept lying around on the couch, which was not his habit. I took him to the children's clinic that we all went to in those days. The doctor didn't say anything to alarm me, but he took a lot of tests and gave me vitamins with iron for him. A day later, Kip was out playing when he came running in with a nosebleed. My kids often got nosebleeds, as did their father, and his mother, so that in itself was not alarming. I could not stop it , however and the color of the blood was too light. I rushed him to the emergency room, after calling his pediatrician. The doctor met me there, he immediately checked him into the hospital. After getting Kip settled and calm. I went back home. I had barely gotten in the door, when the doctor called me and said he was rushing him into Children's Hospital in Boston.

I knew that was not a good sign. The very next day, we were given the terrible news. I could not believe it! Why was God doing this to me! I had lost one child, which is more than a mother can bare, not another one! I think in those days, as self conscious as I was, I honestly believed I was not worthy of having good luck. I believed I was born under a dark cloud, and was destined to be forever plagued with tragedy. When things were going good, I was always waiting for the other shoe to drop, well here it was.

The doctor said, his life span would be about 18 months, in those days that was about all they could offer you. They were just beginning to develop the medicines that now can keep a child with leukemia alive for many years or even forever, but then they did not. He told us not to be taken in by the many charlatans that would offer you miracle cures. He said if anything new came on the market Children's Hospital would have it first. He told us not to neglect our other children while taking care of this one, and not to spoil him or give him his own way just because we were loosing him. I found this all to be very good advice over the next 18 months. At the time I was pregnant again, with a son Duncan who was born six months after Kip got the disease. Kip adored the baby and luckily had some time with him before he passed.

I had been brought up in a Catholic school, and we were taught, when we prayed, that you did not pray for a cure. You prayed for a cure, if it was God's will, if it was not God's will you prayed for a happy death. That's the way I prayed. I prayed if God was going to take him, that he would not suffer, that he would not become swollen with medication, and loose his beautiful hair and that the time he had left would be good for him.

I poured water from Lourdes over him, and I prayed. As hard as the experience was for me, it taught me a lot. I became more spiritual, and stronger physically and mentally. I decided if I could live through this, I could conquer anything! The next eighteen months, were a virtual nightmare. Every time we would plan something, get the kids all dressed up to go some where, Kip would have another crisis. At Easter we were all dressed up for Church, Turkey in the oven, expecting company, when Kip's nose started to bleed and we had to rush into Boston. Then he came down with a terribly sore rash, it apparently had been the result of some infected blood he had received. They had not seen this rash since the invention of penicillin, and he had to get it. To treat it they had to put penicillin several times a day right into his veins. The rash itself was big sores that pained him terribly. He would let no one near him except me, so I had to be in Boston with him and see to my children at home. I was a good six months pregnant or better and I had to carry a six year old around. We got through it, I would keep his mind occupied while the medicine did its job. Two or three times a day they put this medicine into his vein, it took twenty minutes, and apparently it burned or something, because he would scream. I was the only one who could get him occupied in some activity or other to take his mind off it. So I had to be there. Every morning, it was get the other kids off to a sitter or school and drive the sixty miles or so in my impregnated condition to be with him. The rash cleared he came home. When Kip was in Boston, he was always on the eighth floor of Children's Hospital, where all the terminal patients were, but those kids, were so brave they really gave me new courage. I looked forward to seeing them all, they were all like my own kids.

Then after he got home, he started with a new problem, bone pain. He would not walk because it gave him great pain in his joints. I tried carrying him around for a while, but I was getting bigger and bigger and he was a heavy kid. So I got the idea, of pushing his tricycle over to him and making him peddle it. At first he wouldn't but I wouldn't carry him, so eventually he would. The peddling of the bike apparently strengthened his legs and the pain went away.

After that things seemed to look up for a while, he went into remission and for a year or so we had no more incidents and his life went on fairly normally. He went to kindergarten, he played outside with the other kids. He did have to go for visits every few weeks to children's and sometimes he needed a blood transfusion, but he had come to accept that like other kids take cough medicine. He was a really great kid through it all, and I saw some kids who had the disease who so had controlled their parents, it was terrible.

One little girl I remember, She was in a cart, because she was too weak to walk. Her poor mother looked like the wrath of God. The little girl had the biggest bag of candy I have ever seen, she just kept eating it. She whined constantly at the mother to get her this and get her that. The mother went to light up a cigarette and the kid had a temper fit so she put it out. At the rate they were going the mother would be relieved when the child died. She told me she hadn't slept in months!

Kip was so healthy looking at that time, you would have thought the disease had left him, then just as we became confident, it happened.

Three days after his sixth birthday. He was doing great, he had gotten a kite and a new two wheel bicycle. He had been out all day running, playing flying his kite and riding his new bike. He came in tired but rosy and healthy looking. That night he developed a fever. I wound up sleeping with him and giving him alcohol rubs to reduce the fever.

I called the hospital, they told me give him aspirin and bring him in tomorrow. It was the Holy day of the Ascension. The kids were out of school, my stepfather, and Kelly went into Boston with me. By this time, Kip was out of it. He was sleeping very deeply, on the way into Boston, we had to stop at the state police barracks so he could go to the bathroom. We got to the Jimmy Fund Clinic at the Hospital, by this time he seemed to be almost in a coma.

They tried to give him blood and had a hard time finding a vein. He was still answering me if I spoke to him. They decided to do a bone marrow test, just before they took him in, He said to me, Mummy do you see the stars? I thought he was delirious and said Oh yes, I see them. They wheeled him away, five minutes later, his doctor came out. He was all choked up, he put his arms around me, He's gone! he said.

I looked at the doctor and said, Thank God! The doctor looked at me like I was in shock, but I knew he was at peace, I was glad that for him it was over. As tragic as it was, my prayers had been answered. Now, I would have to deal with my own grief, but at that moment I was strong, stronger than I have ever been. I did not cry then, I had too much to do, I had to go downstairs and break it to Kelly and my step dad and then go home and tell my husband! The doctor couldn't believe I was o.k. I assured him I was. I had dealt with this, when they had first told me he was going to die. I had done a lot of my grieving then.

Apparently that night, when he had come in from playing he had somehow contracted meningitis that was what he had actually died from. It took him quickly as I had hoped. I found my stepfather and Kelly, my step dad broke down, Kelly was surprised but she was a little kid she didn't really grasp it. We drove home, and went to his place of business to tell my husband. He completely lost it. He broke down and sobbed for days.

This was his son and heir, he had been named after him and his father, he still had two sons but this one was special.

During the funeral I did not cry, but my jaws were clamped down so hard, I started getting severe head aches. To this day, if I get stressed, that headache comes back, and I had never had headaches before. Other people at the funeral were calling me Jackie Kennedy, but it was just my way. I had learned a long time ago, not to cry at misfortune. From the time my father left me at four, to when my mother left, to Paula's death to now. I was always expected to stay strong for the others, now it was my husband and the remaining children. I could not let them see me fall apart. At night in the darkness, I would sometimes cry as I remembered him.

During the time, that our son was dying, and I was expecting our sixth child, my husband had an affair. His excuse was, I was not paying enough attention to him! When I found out, I was devastated, even though I did not love the man, he had always said he loved me. I had always been a good and faithful wife. He caught me off guard. If it had been any other time, I would have divorced him, but at the time I was pregnant, I had five other children one of whom was dying with cancer. There was no way I could leave or go to work to support us. I was stuck with it, I talked to him, he agreed never to do it again. I told him if I ever caught him near that girl I would leave him or kill them both! I also told him, remember my turn would come! It was an empty threat, but it made him think about it. I thought a lot about divorcing him after that, but it always came back to the same thing. How could I support the kids, and myself for the time being I was stuck. I had no education, no job, four kids now between the ages of six months and nine years old. I would have to wait, but I thought of it often. I thought maybe when the baby went to school. When I would dream of these things, however, I still considered myself to be a very plain, unattractive woman. No man would ever be interested in me. If I got a divorce I would have to be totally on my own to bring up my children, it seemed too overwhelming.

As the children got older, I got more restless. I wanted my own activities and interests. I started collecting antique dolls, and selling Avon. I took a part time job in a restaurant to earn my own money for my hobbies. I only worked a couple of hours a day while the kids were in school. The baby was in nursery school a few hours each day. I decided when he went to first grade I was going to get a full time job. Never happened, the very day he started first grade I turned up pregnant again!

I was disappointed, but I changed the plan, I ran for school committee, and won. I put off the board, a man who had held the position for over twenty years. I continued selling Avon, when the baby was born I just took him every where. I began to defy my husband more and more. The more independent I became the more possessive he tried to be, he accused me of constantly looking at other men. I never did that but he accused just the same. You may think to yourself, didn't they have birth control in those days? Yes they did, but as good Catholics at the time, we were only allowed to use, the rhythm method. That consisted of keeping track of your monthly cycle and only having sex during the time you were not fertile. It worked if you could stick to it, but my husband would say, if I refused him, no church is going to tell me when I can have sex with my wife! I had tried to use birth control pills once, but they were very new at the time, and I was afraid of them.. After using them for a few months, they stopped my periods entirely and I never dared try them again. My husband would not use condoms, and I had seen a diaphragm at the doctor's and just knew I could not use that!! I told the doctor I could never insert that thing in a million years. So it wasn't as if I didn't try. I jokingly told everyone, this baby was a rhythm baby and that one was a birth control pill baby etc. So after Jeremy the last one I got my tubes cut and tied without my husbands knowledge.

Jeremy was born, seven years after Duncan, my seventh baby, my fifth living child. Jeremy had been a terrible pregnancy for me. I was thirty five years old, my body was in good condition, but it had been through a lot. I had every bad symptom a woman can have. Once the baby was born however I was delighted, he was the most delightful baby, he became my constant companion, I took him on my Avon route, and every where.

I became more and more involved in the community, I was not only elected to the city school committee, they appointed me to the regional school committee and the Parochial school committee. I spent a lot of time at school meetings much to my husband's dismay. I made a great reputation as the woman who would fight for your cause, I went places no one before me had gone, from having lunch in the cafeteria's to walking in on certain classes. I investigated the alternative schools cropping up everywhere at the time. I was instrumental in completely changing the make up of the High school, not once but twice during my terms.

I had always wanted to travel, not even having a car, when I was a kid, I always wondered what was on the other side of the hill, the state, the country the ocean. I wanted this for my children as well, I began planning annual trips, whether we could afford it or not! I would plan the trip, figure out exactly how much it would cost. Then I would figure how much I would have to put away out of our budget to do that and I would faithfully put that aside. It might take a year or two but as soon as the money was saved we would go ! We bought a custom van, we took our children to Pennsylvania Dutch country two or three times. They went to Gettysburg, Washington D.C. twice, Williamsburg Va., Atlanta Ga., and Florida twice. They climbed the Washington monument, visited Kennedy's grave, went to the mint, the museums, Disney world and Disneyland, the over-under bridge, and so many places and things. The most exciting trip I took them on, was we spent two weeks on a Greyhound bus, me and my husband

and five children. We got on the bus in Massachusetts on Good Friday, we went cross country to San Francisco, where we spent three days visiting all the sights including the places they had been as baby's. When we got into San Francisco, after three days on the bus, our luggage was missing! Great we hadn't changed our clothes in three days and now we have no clean clothes! Apparently with one of our stops, when we changed buses, it got put on a different bus! We checked into a hotel, I made everybody strip and wrap in sheets and I went to the hotel laundromat to do our clothes. While I was in the laundry, then tried to close it, before I got the clothes dry, but I raised hell and they stayed open till they were done. The following day our luggage caught up with us. One of the things the kids enjoyed in San Francisco was going out to Alcatraz by boat. After the three days in Frisco, we flew down the coast to my father's who had not seen them since they were babies. We spent three days in Long Beach with him. We went to Disneyland and visited relatives. Then back on the Greyhound bus and over to Denver Co. where we had other relatives, we spent three days there, went to the Denver mint and had a great time, then back on the bus and back to Boston. It was a wonderful trip in many ways. Each child kept a journal of his or her experiences. Tod even made a tape we still have and can listen to in his squeaky baby voice. It was a unique trip filled with adventure. We met some very interesting people. In Chicago, while making a pit stop, the police tried to pick up our daughter Kelly, she looked like a runaway and we had to prove it was our daughter to take her with us! In the Midwest, a hippy looking drifter got on the bus, carrying his cowboy boots. He had a long sheathed knife in his belt. Long straggly hair, unshaven, unkempt. He sat down next to Tod. Tod was only ten at the time, and as I said was writing a diary of the trip. The drifter would pull out a butane lighter which was set so a high flame would shoot out. He would strike it, blow out the flame and sniff the butane. I watched him doing this for a while, and spoke to my husband about telling him to stop it. My husband said, I'm not telling that guy anything, God knows what he would do. The drifter kept doing it and it was really getting on my nerves. So I went over to him, I said listen buddy,

I don't want to see you striking that lighter and sniffing it again. He said, what are you going to do about it? I said, well I bought seven tickets for cross country, you bought one for a short trip, if one of us is getting thrown off this bus who do you think it will be? He never lit it again while we were on the bus, he got off a state later. Tod wrote in his diary, my best friend got off the bus today! We met so many fun people, heard great stories, I love riding the bus. It's not the most comfortable way to travel, but it's the most interesting. In a car you always travel highway, in a plane you don't get to see anything but in a bus you go right into the center of the city. A train would be my second choice and that is getting to be more and more desirable.

My husband did not particularly enjoy our trips, he traveled at work, but he would never let me go without him, so he went reluctantly. One time in a hotel room he said to the kids, because they were horsing around, the next time your mother and I are going to leave you at home. I told him, No the next time the kids and I would leave him at home!

Then, I began traveling for the school committee, for the first time I realized other men found me attractive. After our daily conferences, and dinner we would in the evening go into the lounges for conversation and a drink. I was always the center of attention, telling jokes and laughing, I have always had a knack for getting to know people and getting everyone involved. Our table would always be the popular one, and more and more people would seek me out. If there was music, the men would always ask me to dance.

I would never cheat on my husband, but I began to realize that if I decided to go on my own, I would not necessarily have to be alone, or without companionship. This gave me more confidence. I began to realize more, how I had cheated myself getting married so young, for security not love.

I realized even more, how much I was missing by not even being able to be myself. That this little mouse of a person, that lived with my husband was not me, I didn't like her much and I did not want to continue to be her!

When I would return from a trip, my husband would go through my luggage to see what he could find , maybe a clue that I had been unfaithful. At this point I didn't even care, but I did not want to be accused of something I had not done. I needed out of the marriage, but I was still not ready to disrupt my children's lives. I was ever mindful, of the terrible childhood, I had endured and I wanted to spare them that.

If anyone was going to suffer, I had experience at it, I would do it before putting them through it. I resigned myself to my life as it was, but I also was determined to make it more enjoyable. I was going to start trying to be myself when I was out with my husband and not let him intimidate me any longer. For my peace of mind, I contemplated, long range, on probably getting a divorce when the children were grown and on their own. The plan, however, ridiculous made may life worth living and tolerable. I even contemplated having an affair, by this time I was getting offers.

Fantasizing was a harmless and enjoyable pastime. I started paying more attention to my many girl friends. I had at least eight or nine close girl friends, in the same boat as me. They were all brought up more or less the same way, they all had between two and nine children, the average being 3 or 4. They had all been married the same amount of time, some probably had married for love, but most was the same, it was the thing to do in those days. If you were thirty and unmarried you were an old maid!

They were all Catholic, they all did not work, their husbands controlled them and their children. On our street alone there were fifty children between the ages of two and seventeen. The men got together to play pool, they had their bowling and tennis nights, they coached little league, which meant they went to meeting other nights and drank and talked. They spent hours at the Hockey rink or Ball field, when they weren't there, they watched sports or porn. If we were lucky they would take us out on, maybe two Saturday nights a month. Not much different than the life my mother had led. They were slightly better fathers, they did do things with their boy children. Not much with the girls, they were our domain. The wives, took care of the disciplining, the moral upbringing, they were the taxi's for all the lessons, and socializing the children did. The men hardly talked directly to their wives, yet the women waited on them constantly. The men would very seldom baby sit their own kids, it was understood, the women would take them shopping or where ever they had to go. If you did leave them, you heard about it when you got back. Everything they had done the least bit annoying.

I mentioned in a previous paragraph that after the birth of my youngest, I got sterilized without my husband's permission. That is because, he would not hear of such a thing, in fact he got a Vasectomy so that I would not.

You had to have permission from your husband to get sterilized! That so incensed me, that even though he had a vasectomy, I made up my mind I was going to get sterilized as well and no dam doctor was going to tell me that my husband had to give me permission. It took some doing but eventually I got it done. I did not accomplish it for quite sometime however, by that time my oldest daughter was almost in college. I went to the hospital right after my husband left for work in the morning. I got the procedure done , thinking I would walk out of there by noon and be fine by the time he came home from work. By three o'clock that afternoon, I was still coming out of the anesthesia, I finally called Kelly and got her to pick me up. At five o'clock, when he came in the door, I was standing by the stove cooking. He never found out.

The day eventually came, when I could take it no longer. My oldest child was in college, had been for a couple of years, the youngest was only eight but the next one to him was fifteen. My husband was still, reluctantly doing a lot of traveling on his job. When he was away, our house was tranquil and nice, when he was home it was a battlefield. Even the kids were feeling it, we could no longer keep our feelings from them. When he was away, the kids and I would go out to eat, we would relax, have people in. The minute he came home, the stress came with him. He would always want to know everything I did while he was away. I resented telling him so a fight would start. I was fighting for my freedom. One day it all blew up, he had just returned from a trip to Washington state, I had been rehearsing for a benefit show that we put on in town every year, for the hospital. All the people, who were anybody in town, were in it, doctors, lawyers, politicians and their wives or husbands. As a member of the school committee, I was expected to do my part. I had been in it for two years, and I enjoyed every minute of it. This year, I was in the Kick line of the chorus. When he came in from his trip, I was in the bathroom getting ready for the dress rehearsal, I was dressed in a corset type costume for the dance line from Cabaret. He took one look and said, where the hell do you think your going dressed like that!?

You are not going out of the house dressed in that rig! At the time I was a forty-three year old woman, I was highly insulted to be spoken to like I was a child, wife or not. Something snapped and without a moments hesitation, I said. Yes I am, and what is more, I am divorcing you.! It was a little premature, but once the words were out of my mouth, it was like a huge weight dropped off my shoulders. I felt liberated at once, and I knew I had to go through with it ready or not.

Of course he didn't believe me, but he soon found out I was serious. It was a few weeks before Christmas, I didn't want to totally spoil the Holiday.

The following day, I gathered all the children for a talk. They were surprisingly supportive, or most of them were, the two youngest were in shock. They knew it was a long time coming and I think they were sick of the fighting and tension. I had protected them as long as I could. Now it was either take my chances with a divorce or suffocate in a marriage I could no longer endure! While the kids and I were talking about it, my husband was going hysterical, and jumping into the car and driving 100 miles an hour by the house, as if ready to kill himself. It didn't touch me, but the kids were worried about him, so the decision was made that I would leave, and they would all stay in the family home. The older ones would look after the little ones, their lives would stay intact as much as possible. It would give me full freedom to try to find a place, and work.

I told them I would stay home till New Years day. That Christmas was a strange one, the kids all gave me things for my new apartment, (which I didn't have yet). I got towels, and pots and pans etc. I had told them I would take nothing out of the house except my personal things.

On New Years eve, my husband and I went to the church New Years eve party we had always gone to over the years, with all our friends. At the stroke of the New Year I kissed him goodbye, the next morning I left.

I moved in with my youngest sister, Eleanor where I stayed for a month, till I found a job and a little apartment. Eleanor, was the daughter of my step dad, but she and I had always been very close, much more so than my own full sister. I had left home with no job, no education to get one, no experience, and no money. Within that month, I had landed a job in an office down town and got a little apartment. My only furniture was a mattress on the floor. A forty-three year old mother of seven, after twenty-five years of marriage, and nothing to my name, but I felt more liberated and free and happier than I had ever been.

I would miss the kids terribly, but most of them were at the age that I seldom saw them anyway. I lived only a mile or two away and I would see them often. I would not miss the work, the taxiing, the stress. For the first time ever I could do what ever I wanted, whenever I wanted, it was so exhilarating and liberating I could not believe it. Divorce was a rare thing in those days, I had no divorced friends, I did not know any one who had done it. In the eyes of the church and our friends there was something wrong with you if you couldn't keep your marriage together. I was still a very religious and moral person, but in this and birth control I was seriously doubting the churches teachings.

As my married girl friends came to visit, sometimes in a group, sometimes one on one, you could see in their eyes a certain envy. They just loved to sit in the quiet like they were hiding from the world and relax. They would tell me how people were talking about me, and they knew they could not take the ridicule and scorn. It didn't bother me. I knew it would blow over and my life would go on, this time the way I wanted it to. A couple of my girl friends who had been thinking about divorce, one who had been having an affair, changed their minds when they heard people talking about me! You had to be the worst kind of slut to walk out on your husband and children, the man was supporting you, you had a nice car a nice house, what an ungrateful bitch I must be!! I didn't care, I was happy. I had waited all my life to do this, no one was going to rain on my parade!

Freedom is worth it! It's worth anything. Life is too short.

I kept a good repoire going with the kids. The older ones, would take me out to dinner, my oldest son would bring me flowers, or come spend the evening. The girls and I even went out socially or double dated a couple of times. I went to their school functions. The two youngest were the hardest, the fifteen year old felt I had deserted him, it took a long time to get through.

Now almost twenty years later he is finding himself in similar circumstances, what goes around comes around.

Now, I needed to establish a new social life. I had never ever in my life had a date, a drink, or been in a bar or dance hall. I had no idea how to even begin the process. All my friends were married. I started looking in the papers for singles events. The first thing I saw was a potluck supper at the local Y.M.C.A. , that was just down the street from my apartment and it said it was for singles. I made something and went. Most of the people were younger than I but we had a good time talking, one girl was old enough to have a couple of teen age kids, and she was from England. So she became my buddy, we teamed up and exchanged numbers for future socializing.

The following week, Rita and I decided it was time! Our debut, we would drive down route one, and go clubbing! We picked a terribly rainy night.

We had been Non-social long enough! We had no idea where we were going or what we were going to find. Talk about wet behind the ears.

We drove down route one till we saw the first Neon sign flashing, Cabaret.

We drove into the parking lot, which was crowded enough. We

ran inside, it took a while for our eyes to focus in the dark. We sat down at a huge circular bar. A cute little oriental barmaid took our drink order. As we looked around in the darkness we could see there were lots of guys. Great, we'd picked a popular place. There was music playing but I didn't see a dance floor, so when she brought our drinks, I asked her. Is there dancing here. She laughed, only on the stage, I thought that was what you were here for its amateur night! By now my eyes were accustomed and I looked, on this long stage that went all the way across the room, a woman was gyrating to music, half nude, and the guys, tongues were hanging out. Oh my god, Rita and I both spat at the same time. Then we laughed, and asked the barmaid where the closest place was we could go dancing. She told us almost in the same parking lot right next door that there was a little club called the Copa.

We finished our drinks and left. We went next door and it turned out to be one of our favorite clubs for a long time. It was small friendly, and on Tuesday nights they had ladies night. Ladies got in for $1.00 and all drinks for $1.00 for ladies only. It was a great draw, the women came because it was cheap and the men came cause the ladies were there.

As time went on, we discovered other specialty nights at various bars up and down the strip. Wednesday night we went to "The Balcony", Thursday night was "Kaluha" night at the Ashworth, Friday Coastal Singles, Saturday Saugus singles. We went out almost every night, we became some of the most popular girls in circulation. We were not easy, but we dated a lot.

We never went out in the parking lot with anyone, they had to call us for a date. We were out till 1:00 or 2:00 or later every night. Then I got up at six and went to work. Never tired, never had a problem doing my job. It was so great and so new to me, I thrived on the action. Many other single girls as we met them started to hang out with us, because they knew the guys liked us. On Sunday afternoons, we would go listen to Jazz , first at Hampton beach at 3:00 and then on to Portsmouth at 7:00. I never drank, I didn't need to, I had no inhibitions or hang-ups, I could talk to anyone.

Not drinking meant I never had a hang over.

I loved every minute of it, I dated fifty men in the next two years. I was very fussy too, they had to be professional men, they had to have a certain amount of sophistication. I dated a Bass player, for a few months. A man who worked for the F.B.I., a carpenter, an engineer for a railroad, a guy who traveled the world digging huge tunnels, all sorts of interesting and fun men. The ones who wanted to marry me, however, I wasn't seriously interested in, and the ones I was crazy about, didn't want to get serious. Not that I was looking for marriage again, I wasn't but I did want one man that I could have a long-term relationship with. I was still fantasizing about that perfect man who would love me more than life itself.

I was extremely popular, one night for instance I sat down at a club in Portsmouth between two men, one was twenty-five, and one was fifty-four, I was forty-three. By the end of the evening I had a date with each one of them. I went out with the twenty-five year old for about three months, the older man I dated off and on but we stayed friends for quite some time. I eventually fixed him up with a girl friend.

I dressed sexy, because my husband would never let me. I enjoyed making love for the first time, even doing things I had never done with my first husband. I enjoyed, just the joy of conversation, with other adults, and laughing and raising hell! All the bartenders knew me, and knew I drank only ginger ale. Most of the time they didn't even charge me. I always wanted to be in control of my actions, I always wanted to be able to drive safely.

After being single for two years, I met a handsome Sicilian man. I was at the Copa, had just come off the dance floor, he was sitting at the bar talking with a man I knew who was a regular there. I walked over and interrupted them. Sam, aren't you going to introduce me to your friend, I asked. He did and that was it. I didn't let him sit down all night. As we got to know each other better, he kept telling me I do not want to settle down and get married. He had never been married, he was a fifty year old bachelor, I told him no sweat, I was not interested in ever getting married again. I really felt he was the one.

He had a hell of a sense of humor, he was a great dancer, a great conversationalist, and very handsome. All the things, that I had imagined. He dressed beautifully, was very passionate about every thing. We started dating, I broke up with all the other men I was dating, especially one wonderful Greek man who had asked me to marry him.

Eventually, we moved in together, I was beginning to see his bad side, but I was closing my eyes to it. He had a terrible temper, and when he was mad, would swear and scream all sorts of obscenities at me. Sometimes he would have me in tears, but he would come back later all apologies, and I would melt. We lived together for about a year, then he asked me to marry him. I did. He was very supportive of me, he would help me do anything that would make me happy. He helped me buy a coffee shop. He didn't work there except on weekends, I ran it. It became, one of the most successful ever in our area. It was fun, it made me a lot of money. We did very different things there, I was able to use my imagination and do anything I wanted to. It was my business, it had my name on the sign. We played Honky Tonk music, we gave all of our customers their own kazoos. If a particularly popular song we liked came on the tape, we would tell everybody get out your kazoos and everyone would play. Each customer had their own coffee mug which I had picked out for them, the mugs said something about each person. They hung, colorfully, on a huge coffee rack, on the back wall. We wore costumes every Friday, much to the delight of the customers. I wore roller skates everyday while I cooked. The place was popular all over, very tiny diner size but so popular. We made everything from scratch, and gave you plenty. I did this for eight years. Then my husband was offered early retirement from Polaroid. He hated traveling over fifty miles on the highway to work everyday and jumped at the offer.

It was the end of the 80's, the economy was not doing so well, we were beginning to loose money, we could not get good help. I had been through both of my sisters and all my kids. It was time to pack it in. My baby who was now sixteen had been working for us since he was twelve. He spent a lot of time with us. We sold the coffee shop, and moved up North to Lake Winnepesaukee, we took my youngest son with us.

We both found good jobs, me as a bartender, at the local Inn and my husband as a janitor on the second shift at the middle school. It was a beautiful little town, and one of my daughters and grandchildren lived there.

My husband and I although we loved each other very deeply, were fighting more and more. He had a terrible temper, and verbally abused me on a daily basis. He would start swearing at me and calling me names and screaming for almost no reason at all. Because of the problems with my first marriage I would not let him get away with it, I would yell back and so we would have some knock down, drag out battles. The only reason the marriage lasted as long as it did was because we worked opposite shifts. I went to work about six in the morning and got home at two or three. He went to work at two and came home at eleven. After the bartending job, I worked as a restaurant manager, I was getting very bored in the little town. Every weekend my husband and I would travel about forty-five miles to the closest city. We did that every Saturday and again every Sunday. My youngest son worked with me at the restaurant, until he went away to college. He went away to live in Boston. Now I was working double shifts to pay for his schooling. In the summer I made a lot of money, in the winter I starved. The town was utterly boring, I got so I couldn't stand it. Eventually we purchased a condo in Portsmouth so we could stay there on the weekends instead of coming back and forth. Portsmouth was a great seacoast town about fifty miles from where we lived. It was very cosmopolitan, and had everything. We loved going there every weekend. We got along great on the weekends, we had a great time, going to the shows and dancing and eating out. My husband called me his little social director.

At the end of about eight years, I told my husband I could not stand living up North anymore. Also, I could not make a good living, and with college expenses and two houses to support I needed to work more and more dependable. I moved full time to the Condo. He loved our house and his job and didn't want to move, so we decided on an arrangement we would both enjoy. He would live full time at the lake, I would live at the condo, he would come down every weekend and we would spend it together. We would do this until he retired from the school in two or three years.

In the meantime, my husband had a brush with colon cancer, that left him extremely nervous about everything he ate, drank or came in contact with in anyway. Products he worked with etc. He had always been an obsessively neat person, but now it took on another facet. He became so obsessive, he would not get on a plane, or even drive a car in a very busy place. He had been born and brought up in Boston, and had driven there over fifty years. Now, however if we had to take a trip into the airport or go to visit his relatives he was very nervous about driving in there. The worst part is he would not admit he was having these anxieties, so there was nothing I could do to help him.

I would always ask him about vacations, where would he like to go. He would always leave it to me. I would make a suggestion, he would say alright, or I would give him a choice of three places and he would pick one.

Two separate years, I planned a trip I thought he would just love, one was to Italy, he was Italian and had always expressed a desire to see Italy. He gave me the o.k. for it right up until a week or two before we were scheduled to go and would then back out. I took my sister to Italy all expenses paid. The following year, I planned a trip I knew he would enjoy in this country, figuring maybe Italy was too far away. Two of his favorite places were New York and Las Vegas. I planned four days in New York and four in Las Vegas. At the last minute he backed out, I took my son.

He would always say he couldn't get off work or some other phony excuse.

I didn't nag him about it, but I did try several times to approach the subject of his getting help, but he would say he had no problem. He gave them a hard time at work about the chemicals he used to clean, at home everything from the water, to food to what he breathed was suspect. He washed his hands constantly, and got after me to do the same.

Once we were living apart, he in Wolfeboro and me in Portsmouth, it was better but still there. Then one day, after sixteen years of marriage, he asked me for a divorce. He was just about ready to retire again, and I guess he was thinking about having to live with me full time, and wanting control over his own retirement money etc. I was devastated, because this was my retirement too. We had always planned we would retire together, and do a lot of traveling. Now I was fifty-nine, had no retirement of my own. I had run the coffee shop that had given us all the money for our home etc. but I had no retirement because I had worked for myself. Now, he was throwing me to the wolves with no a bit of compassion or concern.

He would have two pensions and his social security, and half the house I had paid for. I would have half the house, no way to make a decent living, no social security to speak of and no pension. I asked him if he was concerned about that, and his answer was, I don't think that because we were married sixteen years, I have to be responsible for you for the rest of my life! Yet he professed that he still loved me , but that we just couldn't live together. He put our home on the market that same afternoon. It was Halloween 1997.

I had no idea what I was going to do. Thank God my youngest son had graduated from College, we didn't have that to contend with. I had just bought my husband a new car, cash the year before. I was driving an old 1992 Cadillac that still had a few month payments on it. I had grown complacent, and a little over weight, because I was content in the thought that my future was secure. Little did I know. I had honestly believed in the past two years we had gotten along a lot better, and were communicating much better. Ha Ha !

That night we were invited to a Halloween party at my youngest daughters. At this point in my life, I could not drive after dark. The glare of headlights just blinded me and I couldn't do it. So my husband asked me if I wanted to go to the party with him. I told him yes, since I had no other way to get there and it was my kids not his. We went to the party and he walked around all night bragging to the kids that he would soon be a single man again. They were flabbergasted but I would not let it upset me. I had a good time, and talked to each of the kids quietly about it during the evening. My children loved him, he had been their father for sixteen years and had a much better repoire with them than their own father did. This was very devastating to them, they had been through it with their father and I and now this. Of course by now they were all parents themselves. Two of them had gotten divorces themselves, so they understood much better than the first time.

I gave myself one day to feel sorry for myself and then I decided to pick myself up by my bootstraps and get on with my life. I could not do anything about this, but I could do something about myself, and I set about doing just that.

My younger sister and her husband had been staying with me, so they would be loosing their home as well. My husband insisted on still coming down every weekend. We only had one bedroom so I made up my mind, that when he came down on Friday night, I would leave till Sunday night when he would go back. Every Friday morning when I would leave for work, I would pack my car with every thing I would need for the weekend. I got a mobile phone so I could still communicate with everyone. I would either stay at my youngest daughter's or my youngest sister's.

So, that's the story, of how I found myself single again at nearly sixty years old. The first thing I had to tackle was, how was I going to be able to support myself for the rest of my life. I had no savings, no diploma, and only restaurant and bar tending experience for jobs.

This book is basically the story of how I did that, and how you can too.

I found, you can continue to re-invent yourself until you die. Your age doesn't matter, unless you let it matter. It doesn't matter how out of shape, or condition you are, unhealthy, fat what ever if you are alive you can fix it. I'm going to tell you how I did it, and will give advice to other women my age in the same boat.

Chapter two:

Ok you're by yourself, you're a middle aged plus woman, you feel very self-conscious. Maybe the reason your husband left you, makes you feel even more self conscious, or insecure. Maybe he left you for another woman? If she was younger, slimmer or prettier, that's even worse ! Maybe he left you for another man! Maybe you got fed up with your lives and his inattention, and left him. Maybe he died. (Those are the only good husbands). Granted this is a very devastating thing to have happen to you, especially at an advanced age, but sitting around for five years, feeling sorry for yourself is not going to change the situation. In fact if your ex and your friends see you sitting around wallowing in self pity and getting fatter and more miserable, after a while their going to think to themselves, he should have left her, look at her she's a mess !

No the best "pay back", is to resurface as this new striking, attractive, self-assured woman. Show him you didn't need him, show him he was holding you back not the other way around! It may seem completely unattainable, but believe me, with just a little, dedication, initiative, and work you can attain it. I did, and I am no more ambitious, or rich, or smart or dedicated than you are, but I am a survivor!

You do not have a minute to spare, give yourself one day to feel sorry for yourself and get over it. You are already middle aged you don't have five years to sit and feel bad. Life is short, and it's your life. He is getting on with his! It is going to take a little while to remake yourself so get to it now!

Make your assessments, stand naked in front of a mirror, get a pad and pen. Be totally honest, but don't fail to notice your good points. This is an honest assessment , not a put down.

When I was in parochial school, the nuns used to tell us, it was a sin not to recognize your talents. That God would hold you accountable for wasted talent. So, honestly look at yourself, What are your good points? Put those down on one side of the paper. Do you have great hair? Pretty eyes, beautiful teeth? Great boobs, good ass, nice feet? There has to be something, nice nails! Can you sing? or play an instrument? Do you have a great sense of humor, can you give a good party? Are you funny? If you have a hard time being truthful with yourself, think about the last compliment you got, what was it on? Ask a relative or really close friend for help with the list. What are your strengths? Now on the other side of the paper put down what you need help on. Are you too fat? too thin? are you the right size but you need toning? Do you have good hair, but its very blah, the color has faded or gone gray and dry? Is the color o.k. but it's too thin and flat. Is your skin bad or damaged from the sun? Have you always been one of those natural women who feel you should leave your hair gray and not wear makeup, but it makes you look old, and plain and invisible?

    If so change your attitude if you want to be renewed. Do you dress, in dark colors all the time? Are your clothes shapeless, ill fitting "fat clothes"?

    Do you wear too long skirts to hide your legs, just because women your age should! Do you wear makeup, is your makeup and hair style the same as it was ten or twenty years ago, or do you update it with the times? Do you dress in a feminine way, do you wear heels ever? Are your upper arms flabby even though you are not fat? Can you touch your toes, can you move easily? How is your attitude? Are you bitter, do you vent that bitterness whenever you talk to someone? Is the sound of your voice, one of whining, or vindictiveness? Every time you get into a conversation with a friend or stranger, do you find yourself talking about your "rotten" husband? O.k. list done?

    If you are a widow, your list will be a little different, but not much. The self-assessment will be the same, as far as your person is concerned. Attitude will be different. You have to work on, not forgetting your wonderful husband, but with keeping him to yourself. Nothing is harder to live up to than a dead spouse. Don't ever compare other men you meet to him. Don't lie to yourself about how wonderful he was. He may have been an angel, but all men have faults. Because he died, don't forget that he was human or no one will ever be able to measure up. I have several friends whose husbands have passed away, when they were alive, they fought all the time like a lot of people, but now that they are dead, they tell you they never fought!

My personal assessment read like this, I was 30 to 40 pounds overweight! I used to be very limber, but now I felt old, flabby, I could barely touch my knees. I got out of breath easily, My hair had been dyed red for years, but now it was getting dull and lifeless, the color was not holding. My clothes were nice, but shapeless. I had to cover my belly, so everything was baggy, elastic waist pants, were more comfortable. I had been dieting for years, buying all no fat foods, but I would diet and then binge on something I had to have. I seldom ate goodies, I bought nothing when I shopped that would tempt me. It didn't seem to matter, I had gained about a pound a year, which is not much but it accumulates. In my twenties I weighed 120, in my thirties 130, in my forties, 140, in my fifties 150 and as I approached 60 I was up to 165 so it was getting worse and I couldn't seem to get a handle on it. My husband had always complimented me and told me I was beautiful so it didn't matter. I hated exercising, I was working in a hotel as a waitress, carrying heavy trays over my head. I was almost sixty, how much longer could I do that? Bottom line, I had to support myself, for the rest of my life.

A scary thought indeed! On my good side of the paper, I was not bitter, I had a great sense of humor. Life had never dealt me too good a hand, so I was used to coping with it. To regrouping every so many years. I had a very positive attitude. I thought of this as a great new adventure. It might be great fun to be single again, if I can get myself looking decent. Right now I felt like a fat, ugly, grandmother, who could barely get out of her own way. My good points, I have beautiful eyes, good teeth, great smile, great legs, good bosom, good rear. That was a starting point. Be realistic about your goals and assets. My self-confidence needed a boot in the ass but I could do it. Above all,

I told myself avoid, negative behavior, nagging, complaining, and gossiping.

Chapter three:

Lets tackle the weight first, the hardest part, or if your thin but need toning you might want to do a lot of this same stuff. Double check your nutrition and exercise.

Are you healthy, do you tire easily, do you feel you have energy and stamina?

It's controversial, but I take about nine vitamins a day, and I have not been sick in over fifty years. No colds, no flu's, no headaches, no sick to my stomach. When our whole work place is down with bronchitis, or flu or colds, I never catch it . If they come into work, coughing all over the place, I spray with Lysol and then take my chances. I add Echinacea to my vitamin routine and double up on my vitamin C , until the crisis subsides. I take every day a woman's vitamin, like one-a-day for women, I take 1000 units of vitamin C, a complex B, an E, 2000 units of Calcium, an A, and sometimes I will add selenium, or billberry but most of the time that is it. I do have allergies, I have to take a shot once a month for that, but other wise I am very healthy. Outside of having seven babies, and breaking my leg, I have never been in a Hospital.

All of my children are into fitness, so I took my weight problem to them. I explained to them, that I don't eat anything I shouldn't yet I could not loose a pound. My oldest son asked me to write down everything I eat.

I went to a dietician and worked out a chart that shows what you need for nutrition every day. We need to eat each day 2 -3 portions of vegetables, 2 portions of dairy, 4 portions of bread, cereal, starches. 1 fat portion, 5 meat or proteins. 2 portions fruit.

Now the catch is what is a portion and it breaks down like this. A dairy portion is 1 cup of milk, or 1/2 cup yogurt. (regular or frozen), A

Bread portion = 1/2 bagel, 1 pita, 1 slice whole grain bread, 1/2 cup rice or pasta, 2 -3 pancakes, 1 cup cereal or 3/4 cup winter squash. A fruit portion = 1/2 cup juice, 1 apple (med.) peach, or orange, 1/3 melon, 1 1/2 cups strawberries, 2 tablespoons raisins, 3/4 cup canned fruit. A meat or protein = 1 oz. meat, chicken or fish, 1 oz. mozarella, 1 slice cheese, 1/4 cup ricotta or cottage cheese, 1 tablespoon peanut butter. A vegetable portion = 1 cup brocoli, cauliflower, asparagus, beans, spinach or turnip or 1/2 cup beets, peas, carrots, V-8 juice, tomato, onion, or 1/4 cup tomato juice or sauce.

Ok so bottom line, your diet and exercise has to be something you can live with. Use what I have told you as a guide. Make up your own diet and exercise program, geared around what you like to eat, and what you like to do for exercise or fun. Only rule, no starving, eat enough, drink water, and do some type of exercise for at least twenty minutes to half-hour every day.

Exercise in some way every part of the body, muscles, abdomen, legs, upper arms, stretch before exercising. Can't wait to see the new you!!!

Chapter four:

The Wardrobe, think sexy, Sexy, SEXY!

"Decide carefully, exactly what you want in life, then work like mad to make sure you get it!" Hector Crawford (1913-1991)

Back to that assessment. Next thing to check, your closets !

Look through them carefully. What is there that needs replacing? Once you loose weight, (if you needed to do that), you will want to wear more flattering, form fitting clothes.

What's in there you haven't worn for more than a year? What is really so worn you should have thrown it out a long time ago, "but its so comfortable?"

Before you actually start throwing, get some current fashion magazines and study them. What's popular? What are the younger people wearing? What would look good on you if you lost what you'd like to ?

We don't encourage a sixty plus woman, to dress like a teenybopper, but you would be surprised how many of their styles can be adapted to look good on an older woman. A youthful style make you look youthful.

What I notice, when I am out at a social or "dress up" gathering, if you look across the room, 90% of the women have on black!

Why? Because they have always been taught it makes you look thin!

While black can be a very sexy, and sophisticated color, it should not dominate your wardrobe. Think about how much you will stand out from the crowd, if everyone else is wearing black, and you're in red!

Go shopping with a close friend, or family member, someone you trust.

Try on all sorts of colors, red, purple, blue's, royal blue, baby blue, turquoise, greens, pinks, from pale to shocking, orange, brown, gray, and even silver and gold. I love bronze! Ask your friend or family member to help you pick the colors that look the best on you, or ask the store clerk.

You don't have to buy yet, just investigate. You may not be the best judge.

For instance, every single time I wear red, everyone compliments me even the bar tender. I now own at least four red dresses. That's your color they always tell me. Don't necessarily believe the first person that says it, but after it's repeated a few times, you'll know. You may have gorgeous blue eyes, royal blue might be outstanding on you, bring those eyes right out!

I have a daughter, that when she was young, had light blonde hair, and she had the biggest brown eyes, I loved her in brown. So take the time, find out what looks good on you, then start buying colors when you shop.

You don't have a lot of money? Can you sew at all, even by hand? You may be able to make over a few of your old things without much skill or money. For instance, this year, the latest fad, is Capri pants. The most expensive ones have fringe, or some kind of trim around the leg. I took a couple of old pairs of pants in my closet, cut them off to mid calf length, and put some inexpensive trim around the legs. You'd be surprised the compliments I get when I wear them. Or pick up a couple of really cheap pairs of pants on sale or at good will and make them over. I also updated an old sundress, I had for at least five years by putting fringe on the bottom and around the neck.

Now for styles, do you always wear long skirts? Yet you have gorgeous legs. Or you always wear short skirts, but your legs are quite heavy? Do you have a great bust line, but cover it because it makes you self-conscious?

Are your clothes too baggy? or too tight? Did you gain a lot of weight, but continue to squeeze yourself into the same dresses? Did you loose a lot and are still wearing your fat clothes? Nothing looks worse than a woman whose clothes don't fit. This is not to say you should not wear figure-hugging clothes, but they need to hug the attractive parts. Again! assess your assets. Notice, honestly, your figure flaws and strengths. If you can't be honest, enlist some one's opinion you can trust, not some one overly critical. Someone honest. You want to dress to accentuate the positive, eliminate the negative, as the song says. Do not go by what your kids say, or a jealous girl friend. Unless your kids are helping you to become more attractive. To most kids, if this is a real change, it's a threat to them. When the transformation is complete, they will love it, but during it, they are afraid to have their mother change. Use your own good judgment,

do what you have always wanted to do, not what you're used to. Don't be afraid to do something entirely different, It's time for a complete overhaul!

If you have a good bosom, show cleavage when you go out. If you have great legs, wear shorts or short skirts. Play up your attributes.

I have always dressed in a sexy manner, but when I got heavy, I started wearing very loose, covering tops. I got up to a size sixteen, my fat clothes. This year for the first time in my life, I was in a size eight. I cannot tell you how that made me feel. I could wear spaghetti straps, and leather dresses, things I had not worn since I was twenty. It felt absolutely great! A couple of my kids, shook their heads at first, but they always compliment me.

I had a job interview last week at the same place my thirty-seven year old daughter works. She called me after I got home and said the guys who work in the office think you're hot! Pretty good for a sixty-one year old woman.

So go shopping, try on the most outrageous things they sell. Try to get comfortable in it. If the mirror tells you it looks good, but your old self-consciousness, wonders if you can pull it off. Just put it on and forget about it. Don't look down, pretend you're in your favorite old black dress. Until the compliments start coming. The first time you wear something entirely different, don't wear it to a family get together, go out to a club or some place where they are all strangers. Get their reactions, family and close friends are not always a good gage. If you're in a new place with new people and you get a good reaction, you'll know you are on the right track.

Now your ready, clean out that closet, if it doesn't fit, if you haven't worn it in a while, if its not your color, if it's not the new you throw it away!

I found a lot of nice new things, at flea markets and the good will. Even accessories, like bags, scarves, and jewelry.

Start trying to wear a little higher heel, Most women our age never wear high heels any more. It's not that we can't, we got out of the habit, our grandmothers never wore sneakers around all the time. They are more attractive, and they do wonders for your legs. Start with just a small heel if you haven't worn them for a long time. Be sure the shoe is very comfortable, but doesn't look comfortable. Try to find a comfortable shoe with style in other words. I have to have a very wide shoe, but I found some of the new shoe store chains, that are really cheap have wide and narrow sizes.

Go up maybe half an inch at a time. maybe a boot. A boot can be very sexy and it gives you a more secure feeling than a strap shoe.

I even went so far as to go for foot surgery, to take off a corn that was paining me for years, so I could wear sexy shoes dancing.

Update the jewelry, I used to wear the biggest earrings around, but right now smaller is in, so I pierced my ears and wear them.

The kid's are wearing glass beads so am I.

How about that hair? Are you wearing a very outdated style? Have you kept up with the crazes? Right now you can't go wrong, it's the unmade bed look. Half up, half down, sticking right up straight, the secret is a good cut.

Look in the mirror, lots of gray? twenty year old style? no luster, dull drab, mousy, no color? Typical old lady style permanent wave, because it's easier to manage? What's the style? Straight and loose or curly and wavy?

Go to a good stylist, even if you can't afford it go at least once, someone with a really good reputation, or a shop with lots of young eager just out of beauty school girls who know what's hot. Ask their advice, not only about a style but also about a color. Do they think you'd make a great blonde, or red head, brunette or some combination. Ask them and go with it, you can always change it, but go with it and decide you will stay with it at least until your next appointment in six weeks. If at the end of that time your not happy with it change it again.. Don't be afraid to be bold. Look through the style magazines they have, ask them could I wear that style? Try it.

Twenty years ago, when I got my first divorce, I went over night from a dull drab dark brown color to a flaming red head, and I mean flaming! Everyone at work told me, your a natural red head, you should have always been a red head! I stayed a red head for twenty years! At first my kids made fun of me. One of my sons called me Flamma for a long time. When it would get drab I would have my stylist brighten it up . Some people would comment on how bright it was but I would always say, You don't understand, Bozo red is what I am going for. That would shut them up.

After this divorce, I wanted to go different again, so after loosing thirty-five pounds, I went to light blonde. I've been that now for a good five years, and I recently asked my boy friends if I should go back to red or brunette? to a man they all said no we love you blonde. It's like being three different people in one lifetime, it's great ! Do blondes have more fun? You bet they do, I can't imagine myself anything else, and neither can my kids or grandkids. The babies think I was born that way.

O.K. its been a struggle, but now we have you in shape, Hair dyed, a striking new style, gorgeous and sexy clothes, Now we need to work on technique and attitude .

Chapter five:

Attitude, Attitude, Attitude!

Attitude, the best word in the English language. It can make or break you.

You can have a bad attitude, or a good attitude. You can enter a room with attitude, you can dress with attitude, you can exude attitude.

Sometimes a prop helps. Do you like hats? Have you always felt conspicuous in one? Try one again. A hat can make a statement, make an outfit, make people look in your direction, make you stand out from the crowd. A flashy little bag, sparkles on your skin, an ankle bracelet all give attitude.

The types of clothing, colors, fabrics all help with attitude, so choose with what you want to say in mind. A leopard garment says something, suede or leather, zebra, pony any animal print. Snake is big right now. I wear a lot of animal prints. My sunscreen has sparkles in it.

A massive gold bracelet, a toe ring, fringe, feathers, beads, chokers, all say something. A cowboy hat gets a lot of attention, a Rod Stewart hair do. Men love chokers, no matter what your kids or girl friends say. I worked with a lot of twenty year old girls, I was in my late fifties at the time. They always asked my opinion about clothes and accessories, especially if they were going out on a date with a new guy they wanted to impress.

The average twenty-year-old wears little or no makeup, their hair is usually straight down and no style, or if it's naturally curly just wild and bushy all over the place. The dressiest thing they own is black dungarees or maybe a mini skirt, and those ugly clunky shoes. I would always suggest they get a dress, and high-heeled shoes of some sort.

They can still be platforms or clunky heels if that's what's in, but high-heeled sandals with a strap turn on a guy. I always suggested a choker, even before they became fashionable, as I think they are right now. At first they would make fun of the idea, but every time they tried it, it was successful. One girl was going out on a hot date for valentines, she wanted to make a big impression. She had been going out with this guy for a few weeks and he had been wonderful to her. She wanted to do something great for him to impress him.

I picked out a great cozy intimate restaurant for her, and told her to dress up sexy. She said the dressiest thing she had was black jeans, I asked her if she had a red sweater, she did. I told her to wear a choker, and if she didn't have one to tie a narrow red satin ribbon around her neck. She thought I was stupid but she tried it. The date was a big hit, he loved the choker, it had been an absolute turn on to him. That was three years ago, I just got an invitation to their wedding. I haven't worked with her for two years, but I brought her back a choker when I went to Spain.

A month ago, I was at the singles. Two girls walked in wearing cowboy hats. The place was mobbed. At first all the girls around the bar made wise comments about them, but no one could keep from looking at them. Within a half an hour they were totally surrounded by eligible males.

Another lady that I know, she is a good-sized lady, she always wears a black felt hat, pulled right down to her eyebrows. There is nothing else about her that is significant. She usually wears a black dress, or pants. She is just average looking but she is very popular, always out there dancing. She does have a great sense of humor, which helps, but any other lady her size would get no attention, the hat makes her unique.

Anything, that singles you out from the crowd, gets you noticed. That is not to be confused with looking ridiculous, or causing a major scene of some sort. We are talking subtle, attractive, but outrageous.

Then you need a good mental attitude. My fiancée always says, walk in looking like you just had it, and couldn't care less if you never had it again.

Don't ever look needy. Someone may jump on needy, but they'll just use you and walk away.

My way is, walk in like a panther, stalking his prey. When you enter a room, walk tall, chest out, head high, tummy sucked in. Walk one foot directly in front of the other, slowly carefully, don't rush. Slinky, make a statement, like you own the room, pretend your a model on a runway. Slither, slink, if you think you are gorgeous everyone else will think so too.

Even if you really feel unsure. Having second thoughts about what you picked out to wear, self conscious about your hair, what ever, forget it and walk like a queen. Smile, smile, smile, even if you feel like shit. Smile all the time. Laugh out loud, when you hear something funny. Laughter is contagious, people always comment about my laugh and my sense of humor.

I knew you were here, I heard you laugh all the way across the room. (and they sought me out).

Attitude is the ultimate cool, how do you become cool? First of all you have to get rid of the stress. Now you say to yourself, Oh sure just like that.

I know it's difficult, I know it's almost impossible to stop thinking about all the things that stress you. You can if you want to, help yourself to lessen the impact of these thoughts on you life. You can come to grips with what stresses you, and lessen its harmful effects, so no one will be able to tell your stressed. Think about what you are stressed about, is it job, kids, wife, ex wife, ex husband, money, future, what?

Lets take your job for example, (I will get into jobs more in depth in another chapter), but for now. Is your job causing you stress? Do you hate your job? or is it just certain things at your job that if they were not there you would be very happy with your job? Determine which. If you hate the job, work on your resume, then get them out there, everywhere, go to a headhunter. Just the fact that you are looking will lessen your day to day stress, because you will be saying to yourself, just a little while longer. If its just something at your job, a co worker, unrealistic expectations from your boss, anything . Make an appointment with your boss, and let him know, what's bothering you. Let him know that if this problem was corrected you would be a much happier camper, and he would get much more production out of you. Most bosses would be happy to be able to alleviate a problem. If that doesn't work, have a meeting with your co workers, make it a bitch session find out if they have similar gripes and take them enmass to the boss.

If nothing works, go back to the resumes. Sometimes the mere act of talking it out, makes you feel so much better you can go back to work and the stress is gone.

The exercise I do in relating to stress goes like this. No matter what the problem is. I always imagine, what is the worst thing that could happen? Then I think about how I would handle that, in a realistic manner. Once I work out in my mind how I would handle the very worst scenario anything else in easy.

If it's your kids, remember you are the parent. They may be forty years old, thirty, twenty but if they are giving you a hard time, making fun of you, telling you how you should live, trying to get you to baby sit all the time, working on your guilt. Think of them as if they are still four years old, or ten years old. How would you have handled it then? Do the same now. Let them know, you are the parent, you will make your own decisions, and you expect their loyalty, and respect and you will accept nothing less. With discipline, its effectiveness is also attitude. If you say it with authority, ending on a firm tone, not a question in your voice they will not question you. Children are always going to act negatively to any major change they see in mom, at first. However, once they see the new you, and see your success, they will compliment and be very proud of you. No child or grandchild wants to see their comfortable, fat, gray haired mom or grandma, turn into an attractive, sexy looking woman. Do it, not for them for you, and two years down the road, after you've adjusted your life they will be bragging about you to their friends. Its good for them too, remember how they always say, if you want to see what your wife is going to look like when she's old look at her mother. Well my girls tell me their boy friends comment on that, and say if you look as good as your mother when your past sixty I will be happy.

Is it your ex that is causing you stress? Remember, he is your ex ! He has no more rights over you than the stranger you meet on the street! Treat it that way. If a stranger threatened you, or intimidated you, you would reciprocate, take out a restraining order, whatever to put a stop to it. Do the same with an ex. Pretend it's a stranger, would you put up with what he is dealing out? He still thinks of you as his possession, let him know your not.

Be above his anger as much as you can be, to keep yourself from being stressed. Look down your nose at him, rather than allowing him to rattle you or get all worked up, he thrives on getting you stressed. If you need to take him back to court do it, and you don't need an attorney, you can go to family court and file anything you need to on your own, learn how to do it. It will save you thousands of dollars. If he is just making mean comments, remember its jealousy based and ignore it. The more gorgeous and self-sufficient you become, the more comments he will make. Just smile and say, you think so? If you turn into a knockout that turns men's heads, he will be kicking himself for letting you go. One night my ex husband came to the singles, where my fiancée and me hang out with our friends. We brought him into the fold and introduced him to everyone, after a couple of weeks one of the guys said to him, your wife is gorgeous why did you let her go? He just turned red and said, we get along better this way. Not long after that he stopped coming.

Anything else that stresses you in your day to day living, slow down take a look at it, ask yourself why am I letting that stress me? Sit down put your feet up, have a cold drink, relax take a look at it. Remember, "It's only a Movie", if you can look at life that way you can find humor in your daily drudgery. Life can be a whole bunch of wonderful adventures, if you tell yourself that everyday, you can't go wrong. As I tell people, everyday I wake up on this side of the dirt, I'm one step ahead! Life is very short, remember that when your allowing time for depression you're wasting time, experience as much as you can. Be willing to try anything even if it's a little scary to you.

I went hot air ballooning this year it was fantastic, I'm hoping to go sky diving next year. I travel to Europe and over seas as often as I can. I heard a great line today on a car commercial, it was, "remember the compliments you get, forget the insults." That's great advice, it will create great attitude. All those corny sayings, "When life gives you lemons make lemonade", are true. We just have to live by them.

Finances what stresses you? Make a budget, live by it. Work on paying off your credit cards, even if you have to sacrifice a while to do it. Take in a roommate, get an extra job just for a short time. I eat healthy but very cheaply. I go out a lot but take advantage of every bargain I can get. Use coupons, take your lunch. With my share of the money I got from the sale of our communal home, I bought a condo. It's not the most luxurious one I could find, but it was in my price range. It's totally paid for and I don't have to worry about someone throwing me out of my house. When my fiancée moved in, I thought maybe we should buy a bigger one. I decided no, we would rather use our money to travel, this is fine and comfortable and convenient. I buy a lot of new clothes to go with my new life for both of us. I never pay full price, I buy through the catalogs, or on sales or at discount stores and we are the best-dressed people at the singles. If you're a woman and you look good and you get out there, you don't have to worry about entertainment. The men will pay for everything. Before I was engaged, I was out to dinner every night, with a different sexy man. Always to a nice place, great conversation, dancing, anything I wanted even long week ends and trips. Now some women I know are going to disagree with that, they're going to say, you should pay for yourself, you should not use your sexual wiles to get what you want. Bull, a man got you into the situation your in let him help you to get out. Of course this is all your own decision do what makes you comfortable.

O.K. Attitude to reiterate, you need to relieve the stress, you need to be able to say honestly, I am great. If you have to fake it for a while do it. Don't keep looking in the mirror. When you are getting ready to go out, get yourself to your most attractive. One last look in the mirror, full length, assure yourself you're gorgeous, then don't look again. Don't sneak peeks in the reflection of the car, or the car mirror. From the time you leave the house walk as I told you imagining you are the most beautiful woman in the world.

A panther on the prowl, straight tall, breasts out , stomach in, slowly provocatively. Always walk that way even to the super market, it will become a habit. Don't go out of the house without following that regime, even if you are in dungarees. Don't ever sneak out for a moment to the mailbox or the market, in some horrible outfit or no make up. That's when you will see the man of your dreams, or your most hated woman friend! Never leave the house in sweats, even if you're going to the gym! Find a cute, short set or gym clothes that are attractive. Don't ever go out without your hair and nails groomed, you never know who you'll see at the dumpster. If you're having a bad hair day, go back to the hat, even if it's a cute baseball hat. I have a denim baseball hat that says "Killer" that my fiancée got me. It covers a multitude of sins. I also have a sequin baseball cap for dressier moments. Attitude, attitude, attitude, Smile, smile, smile.

Chapter six:

Time to make new friends, and influence people

Live every day as though it's your last. One day you'll get it right.. Zig Ziglar

Ok you've lost weight, or at least are trying. Your hair is a new and exciting and youthful style. Your body is toned or on it's way, your hair is a new brilliant and exciting color, You are experimenting with new makeup and clothing, you are trying to walk in high heels again, and your working on your stress level, and social skills.

Now how do you begin this new life? How many girl friends do you have that are around your age or in your life style? Old girl friends you grew up with, old girl friends you were chummy with during the raising of your children, from your old neighborhood. Did you hear some of them are recently divorced also. Maybe their are women in your work place that are recently divorced or widowed and chomping at the bit to change their lives but don't know how to. How about single older women that for whatever reason never married. Women who may not really be your friends but would love to get out for an evening and do something. Befriend every body.

Talk to people at work, find out if they are open to going out. Talk to them about how you would like to go out and socialize but have no one to go with. Search them out till you find a few that you feel you can socialize with. Get a little group of you and go together at first. Sometimes it's easier with companions. Or you can start with just one, like I did with Rita after my first divorce. I was more fortunate after my second divorce there were many more divorced or single ladies, which was surprising to me. There were more women divorced when I was in my sixties, than there was when I was in my forties. A sign of the times I guess. I met a group of ladies at work that went out every Friday and Saturday night to a singles, at a big hotel ballroom about forty five miles away. They car pooled and their were between four and eight of them every week. They were kind enough to include me. Up to this time in my life, I could not drive at night, especially to a place I had never been. My eyes were affected by the glare of the lights, especially in bad weather. I couldn't see a thing. Whenever I went out I always had a girl friend drive. Now that I was single I was going to have to somehow over come that. I started by having a really good eye test and check of my contacts and glasses to be sure my vision was as good as I could get it. Then I started driving only on divided high ways where the cars were more lanes away. I got U.V. approved sunglasses. and I would train myself to look away from the glare.

So in the beginning I invited myself along with the girls, and didn't offer to take a turn car-pooling. One of the girls would always pick me up. Then we would meet the others at a designated spot within an eight-mile radius, and all go in one car. Luckily at the beginning one of the girls did not mind driving and she did it a lot, we chipped in for gas or paid her way into the dance. Eventually I learned the way and took my turn, looking back on it now, I'm sure it was a form of anxiety because I am never troubled by it now and drive all over after dark.

The first time I went with them, it was winter, and I wore slacks and a sweater and fashion boots. When I got there, I was impressed with the place. I had not been in a singles for over twenty years. It looked like a wedding hall, lots of big tables for eight or ten people. It had a very large dance floor, and two bars, and a table with snacks. The bars were service bars, not the type you could sit at, and there was always a line of guys at the bars.

You could meet someone standing in line. There was a D.J. it cost $8.00 to get in, but that included the appetizers. You need to get there early to get a decent parking place or a table to sit at.

Most of the men, came late and stood in double and triple lines in front of the appetizer table. That way when a woman would come over for a snack she would have to walk through them and they could get a good look.

Most of the men were too shy to approach a table full of women, unless they first saw you dancing with other men. They still had a hard time coming up to a full table of women. They worry more about rejection than we do, and it's especially humiliating in front of other women. For this reason I never refused anybody at least one dance. If they become annoying then you can humiliate them. If after one dance you quickly say, thank you, excuse me and leave the floor they get the message. If you can summon up the courage the best way is for the lady to ask them, unless you are a real dog, they will be great full and dance with you all night, and usually ask for your number, and you have done the picking. If you're afraid to ask, just non-chalantly wander over by the buffet table and stand near the one you like, usually you can start a conversation.

Men always stand by the bar, buffet table or the ladies room, hoping you will notice them on your way by. They are by far more self-conscious than the women are. Of course the jerky looking guys will always ask, they must have read my book on attitude, because the real homely, stupid, unkempt, bad in any way ones, always have the most confidence, God knows why.

Use them, dance one dance with them if they ask, the other guys will notice, and it will give them the confidence to ask you. Never unless you have had a bad experience with a guy, refuse anyone. If the other guys see you turning anybody down they will never ask you. Dance at least one, be polite, smile, listen carefully to the music, because a D.J. tends to run one song into another. As soon as you hear the music change to another tune, thank him, excuse yourself and he will get the message. The other guys will notice and know you are approachable.

This works the same, if you see a guy you like, and after dancing with him change your mind for some reason do the same thing. Listen when the music changes to a new song, thank him and excuse yourself from the floor. Most disc jockeys play sets of four or five songs you could be up for a long time if you don't do that, and with someone you don't want to be with that could be a real long time. If you have gotten the courage to ask someone to dance and it doesn't work out, immediately ask someone else so the first one won't zone in on you.

Or he might keep asking if he didn't get the message. Sometimes you have to say no, but only if a guy is really persistent after you've given him the message. If you spot someone you want to dance with and you are too chicken to ask him. There are ways to get him to ask you without leaving your seat. Focus on him, keep glancing his way, if he looks at you lock eyes and smile. Wait for him to smile back then, drop your eyes and look up and smile again coyly. If you do this long enough he will come over and ask you, or if you are getting the right signals and he doesn't come walk over and say Hi and start a conversation. There are lots of ways to start a conversation, the most used are, Is this your first time here? , Come here often?, I love your tie, or shirt or something, "wow, Quite a crowd tonight huh?, Music's a little loud huh, hard to talk.?, then keep it going. Do you come here often, oh its your first time, mine too. Do you live nearby? ....

If he doesn't get the hint, ask him to dance, or ask if he likes to dance. If he is not interested, say Nice meeting you and leave. Wait a while and try someone else. Don't be discouraged and don't take it personal. Remember there are a lot of confused, hurt and bitter people out there. Even though they are there they may not be ready for a relationship or even a dance. Along with the sweet lonely ones, a lot feel they have been hurt too many times to take chances and are very ,very cautious . The second or third time you meet the same person he can be entirely different. Remember you have to kiss a lot of toads, to find a prince.

There are a lot of different kinds of singles out there, and you really need to experience them all, to find the right situation for you. Everyone is different and different set ups work well for different types of people. Give each place a fair chance, go at least three times, if you are not having a good time try something else. I have gone to the exact same place three or four times in a row and had an entirely different time each time. It depends on the crowd. Sometimes the men outnumber the women, sometimes its the other way around. Sometimes everyone seems very friendly sometimes very aloof, you never know. On certain holidays there are always more men than women, for instance Christmas night. Not Christmas Eve, but Christmas night. A Friday night is always different than a Saturday night. Singles in the suburbs are always different than in the country or city. I find men in the country or suburbs are much more apt to ask you to dance. The women in the country or suburbs are not as attractive and more apt to be overweight. The people are friendlier, and more genuine. In the city the women are very sophisticated, all have artificial nails and are skinny, they dress better their hair is always coifed. The men are also more sophisticated, and better dressed, more professional, more on top of things, but may be harder to get to know, more jaded. They talk more than they dance. Usually more money.

There are exceptions to this, some of the more cosmopolitan, towns or suburbs are very affluent, yet the people will have the qualities of small town living. You should try out every singles within a sixty-mile radius, to find the ones you like.

Singles have a bad name. Everyone, including my children, call them, "Meat markets", bars etc. They are not that way. You need to go to find out, it's more like a club. Like belonging to the Elks or the Moose only with all single people. Some are more attractive than others, but basically they are just get togethers for single people, usually between the ages of 30 and 70.

People just like you, single lonely, looking for friendship and companionship. I have met as many great women as I have men, and some have become my best friends over the past three years. I seldom see the first group of women I went out with anymore, they have all met someone and moved on. I have met a whole new group of extremely nice people, and even though I am engaged, I keep going because we would greatly miss seeing these people each week. My fiancée feels the same way.

Another singles we go to regularly, is about 38 miles away and closer to the city. The set up is different, and perhaps is more conducive to meeting people. It has two bars, bars you can sit at. One is up four stairs off the dance floor, almost like on a stage, with a railing people can stand and lean over looking at the dance floor, the other is on the ground floor to the left of the dance floor but near the buffet table. This singles, costs $5.00 apiece and serves a hot buffet.

The men especially like this because they don't like to cook. The dance floor is very large and the place can comfortable hold 500 people, it is open every Friday and Saturday night. Their is another one about 45 miles away same type of set up, same price but its only open on Tuesdays nights, and you would not believe the crowd they get on a Tuesday night. Again you need to get there early to get your favorite seat, we have been going so long the bartenders sometimes save our seats. We always sit at the same place at the bar and all of our friends know just where to find us. In the middle of the evening we turn our stools around back to the bar and just entertain all the people who have gathered near us. There are also small tables scattered around the dance floor, but its harder to get to know lots of people seated at a table. As the evening progresses the men stand in rows of four or five deep between the bar and the dance floor making it difficult to get through to get to the floor, but that's why they do it. They get a good look at all the women as they squeeze through.

Same rules as at the other place as far as asking men to dance or giving them the eye so they will come over. The only difference is when your seated at the bar if you smile at a guy across the room his excuse to come over will be to get a drink and he will lean across you to get the bartenders attention and start a conversation that way. I have met dozens of men this way.

If you are sitting at the bar, talking with all your friends and people who come by, and laughing out loud, they will notice you and slowly wander over to be included in the fun. Our area of the bar is always crowded with people who have gotten to know us and want to be included in our group. Get to be friends with the bartended, its always fun when a guy has been standing behind you for half an hour trying to get a drink, and you offer to help and you call the bartender right over by name and get the drink for him.

In two short years, I have become the most popular person in at least three or four different singles. Everyone wants to sit with us, talk to us or be included in our group, I feel like one of the jocks when we were in high school. We give out a lot of advice to newly divorced people or people who have been divorced for a long time but are not coping well. I was one of the misfits in high school, I know how it feels so we try to help these people all we can.

The very first time I went to this singles, in Danvers, I went by myself. I had not been there before, I had heard about it through the grapevine. I had a small fight with a guy I was going out with at the time, and just took off and wound up there. I sat at the third seat at the bar, the first two seats were taken by two tough looking guys who looked like they belonged in the Mafia. When I smiled at them they just growled at me. I didn't let it intimidate me.

I had a pretty good time, I met a few people but I felt it was a little "clicky". The following week I went back again, again alone. This time I met a few more people and had a better time. The third time I went, I got there early and sat in the first seat at the bar where these guys usually sat. They came in and sat in the next two, they gave me a dirty look I smiled prettily and asked if they wanted my seat they growled no. Since then that has been my seat and we have become great friends. Slowly but surely we met more and more people, I met my fiancée there and now we are the most popular people there. I never went there without meeting at least two nice guys a week, they always asked for my number and I dated maybe a dozen or so before I met Jim.

Now this next thing, I believe is the one thing that causes more misunderstandings between men and women than any other thing. Men take the phone numbers of any attractive women they meet. Its like the gun notches on the belts of the cowboys. They are not necessarily going to use them, but the other guys always ask them, did you get any numbers? Its stupid but its a guy thing. Now they might use them, but it may be awhile. The guy with the most numbers at the end of the night is the winner, especially if one of the numbers is a girl they are all hot for. Of course the ultimate trophy is to find a woman who will take you home that night, but if that can't happen a number is the next best thing. Or better yet, a "parking lot job", which is a quickie or blowjob in the parking lot. Now to us girls this stuff sounds gross, but to guys its not. Don't be shocked just be aware. I wouldn't even let a guy walk me to my car, until I was going fairly steady because I didn't want anybody to think I was going home with somebody.

I almost never went home with anyone, they had to call me for a date. Now here is where the disagreements come in. A girl figures if a guy takes her number he will call her at least during the next week that seldom happens. So the following week they see each other at the singles, and he hasn't called! The shit hits the fan, why didn't you call me? Out come all the phony excuses, then they get arguing. The fact that a man takes your number is not a promise to call, after you give it to him forget it. He will call sooner if you don't mention it. If you get into it with him the number goes in the trash. Many numbers wind up in the trash anyway, or the laundry, in a pants or shirt pocket that's hanging in the closet, in a suit jacket pocket he will find at the next wedding. Point being, if you want to be popular, don't ever ask him why he didn't call. If he sees you and says, hey I'm sorry I didn't call, you say, no big deal, they're a dozen more where you came from. You can bet he will call during the week, unless he honestly lost the number. If a man took your number, he finds you attractive, he may need to get to know you better at the dances before he actually asks you out. He may be waiting till he has the money for a really good date, he may be in a relationship he is trying to get out of. He could even have been so drunk at the time he forgot he took it. In which case he will probably ask for it again. Bottom line give him the number and forget it, if he calls its a bonus.

Always be busy at the singles talking to other men, don't wait for him, make him work for you. Every man wants what someone else has, and they are not used to someone who doesn't "act like a typical woman". I never ever hassled a guy about not calling , I always had a few on the string and sometimes I was glad they didn't call, I didn't have the time.At one point I was dating as many as seven guys at one time, and I always let them know it. Not to brag or rub their noses in it, but for centuries, guys have done that, and the women always wondered if they were the only one.

Guys think it's cool to have a lot of beautiful women, but if a woman does it she's a slut! Well your not, if you can fit it into your life, do it. I never told another guy, details about my dates with others, but I let them know I was seeing other men and intended to continue to do that. For some reason, when the average guy knows he's not your one and only, he falls all over himself trying to be the best. He's more attentive, more polite, spends more money, takes you on better dates, and if your having sex, tries to be the best at that.

Often they would show up at the same place, two or three of them and all hang around trying to get my attention. But, I had a rule, if you didn't bring me, you don't own me and I will have a good time with every body. I even introduced them to one another, and today they all know each other.

Very often, after I became popular, I would still meet an average of two new guys a week. When they would ask me out, unless they were extra special, and I wanted to give up an old one, I would say sorry my program is full. I'm dating four or five guys now, I don't have time for any more. They would be devastated, and would keep asking me week after week. Do you have any room on your program for me yet? They would continue to ask me to dance and be as charming as they could, hoping I would change my mind.

My point is, I am not overly attractive, there were always much prettier girls at the singles than I. They didn't know how to play it, they didn't know how to handle guys, they didn't know how to pick out the good from the bad in the first place. I'm not better, I'm smarter, I do it differently than most of the women. I don't get upset if a guy doesn't call, I don't get upset if he doesn't respond immediately, everything is a game. It's only a movie. Relax, enjoy, If you want to stand out from the masses of single women everywhere, you have to have a different agenda. If you are the same you will sit there alone. Men hate women who cry in their beer, they hate women who constantly put men down, they hate needy, whiney women. Always be up, they don't want to hear how your ex screwed you in the divorce. If they do they will ask. They don't want to hear your ex is a terrible father, How you have to do everything. Don't you think that reminds him of his own wife and kids? He can probably hear his ex saying the same thing, you certainly don't want to sound like his ex ! He doesn't want to hear how terrible your life is and how you need someone to help you. Don't tell him you need someone to fix your car, or repairs around your house. If you find a nice guy that will be a bonus, but no guy wants to start a relationship that way.

Be the ultimate, independent, desirable, sexy woman. You don't need a man for anything, but you might want one. Make him think he needs you. Listen to his every word, be there for him. Let him do things for you. Expect him to idolize you and he will. Let him open the door, he will fix your car, or house, but in his own time, at his own suggestion, to please you.

Suggest places you would like to go, but notice if he seems to have a lot of money or a little. If he doesn't seem to have too much, suggest places you would like to go or things you would like to do that don't cost anything. Like, I would love to take a ride up the mountains this weekend and have a picnic on the way. Or I love walking on the beach, or going to a movie.

There are a lot of really nice guys out there that are paying out a lot of child support or alimony that can't afford two or three meals out in a fancy restaurant each week. If you are really attracted to him, it could make the difference between you and some other girl getting him. Be understanding, cook dinner for him once in a while. Look in the paper for places to go, craft fairs, chowderfest's, hometown activities. Cook popcorn at home, and sneak it into the movies. It can be fun, and save him $10.00. Drink soda once in a while instead of the real expensive drinks.

On the other hand if you know he has money, don't settle for just nights at his place, or cheap dates. Some of the richest men I know are the cheapest, and you want to know that right up front. There is a guy we all know who goes to the singles. When he meets you, he will take you to see his house, which is one of the most gorgeous I have ever seen. That's it, after he's shown you his cars and house, he expects you to come see him there when ever he wants, but he won't take you out or spend a dime. Needless to say, word has gotten around and he is a pretty lonely puppy.

There are also a lot of other ways to meet people, and get dates, other than the singles clubs. There are the singles magazines, and brochures, you can usually pick up at your local super market. These are very informative, they not only have adds for single men and women , but they also have long lists of places to go, travel clubs, parents without partners, skiing groups every possible thing you can imagine. You can look it over and pick out activities that appeal to you and go there. The travel clubs book only singles trips. There is also Internet dating, dinners etc. Don't be afraid to try any of these things, just because somebody tells you it's not a good idea. It can be as safe as going out and meeting someone if you use common sense. I have tried them all, and have my own opinions but one is as safe as the other if you do it right. The rule is , do not give out anything but your phone number. Not even your last name. Meet for the first time in a very public place. Take your own car. Make a date the first time just for coffee, or a drink in case he's a loser your not stuck for a whole dinner or evening. If he seems real nice at the first meeting, meet for a second time, but keep the same rules.

Maybe in between you can talk on the phone. When you talk on the phone, prepare your questions ahead of time, in such a way that you will get to know a lot about him. Find out how many times he was married, what happened. How many children, who has them, what does he do for work?

Is he from a big family? Do they get along, is he close to his folks, his siblings.? All these things tell you something about him, other than the answer to your question. Ask them in a nonchalant way, don't rapid fire them at him, like your interrogating him. I met a couple of nice guys through a dating magazine. I prefer to meet face to face at a club, but for some people its better not to. If you're shy or unattractive, or want someone to get to know you by phone or computer first. You can call or write several men that sound good to you by their add. They will call you back and that's all their is to it. If they get a lot of answers you may be in competition with a lot of other women. If that's the case, he may take you out then you won't hear from him for a couple of weeks while he tries the others, but may come back.

The first man I met through the singles magazine, was extremely attractive, there was definite chemistry on both sides. We went out a few times, but after about a month, he dropped me for an old flame that had come back into his life. He was the only guy who ever dropped me! The second man I met through the singles magazine, was tall, blonde attractive, but he had a hair do strictly from the 50's and 60's a cross between Elvis and Englebert. I could not get by that, he was very nice, polite quiet, attractive. At the end of dinner I told him, I like you a lot but I can't get past your hair do. I did not go out with him again. I like my men to look stylish and up to date. Sophisticated, not country, or biker.

A really neat way to meet men and even other women, for friendships is the dinner parties they have now for that. You are matched up by computer, or by interests, and likes and dislikes. The hostess invites twelve couples, six girls and six boys. It costs you about $60.00. You get a five-course meal, and drinks. You all sit around a big table and after each course the men move their seats to the next woman. Over the course of the evening you get to know everyone. You give out only your first name, and you tell the hostess at the end who you are interested in. She will ask the man if he would like to go out with you and if so will pass on your number. If he would not she will tell you. You can like all six if you want or one or two. My daughter met a man a couple of years ago at one of these dinners and they have been going steady ever since. All of the people at the dinner are compatible to you. In ages, interests, music activities etc. If you do not meet someone at the dinner you like. you will be invited free of charge to another one until you do meet someone.

You can't meet someone unless you are out there looking, and nowadays there are so many singles, at churches, on the radio, in your evening paper.

Try everything, don't get discouraged , you will find your thing, their are singles cruises, and even singles apartment buildings and condos.

Chapter seven:

How I did it

When I hear somebody say, "Life is hard." I am always tempted to say, "Compared to what"?...............Sydney Harris Newspaper columnist

O.K. Now that we've given you the basic formula, I will take you back to my personal journey, over the past two years. It may help you to realize the basic types, and mistakes that we all fall into. Besides I would never tell you to do something I had not tried myself and found that it worked.

Remember, I am no smarter, no prettier, no skinnier than you. I have all your faults and then some. I learned how to handle them and what to do about them.

First of all, I have always been, a very clumsy person. If someone is going to trip over their gown and fall down the steps, it will be me! Anyone who knows me well, will tell you that. I have taken some of the most fantastic falls you have ever seen. I am totally untalented, but I have a great sense of humor and can laugh at myself. I am a funny person, and can often have a whole room in stitches, telling stories about my escapades, or jokes.

The only way I get through life, is sheer determination, stubbornness, and grit. I have terrible luck, I have never won anything, I am always hurting myself, walking into something, tripping over something, or hitting something. I burn myself on my curling iron every time I use it.

One Halloween night, I had to baby sit my grandchildren for my youngest daughter. She had to work that night, and she wanted me to take them trick or treating. My daughter works at a Hospital and she wanted me to pick them up there. They had been out with their father for the day and he was dropping them off there. I got to the Hospital, and went into the reception area. As you entered the Hospital, you passed through two huge glass, electric doors. The entire wall, surrounding the doors, was also glass, from the floor to the ceiling. I went up to the receptionist and asked her where the respiratory department was as that was where my daughter worked. While she was looking it up, I glanced up and saw my grandkids outside with their father. Without thinking I ran toward them, smashing into the glass wall, beside the door. I hit it full on with my face!

The entire wall came crashing down to the floor. It didn't break it just fell over! I gasped, touched my face to be sure I wasn't bleeding then went outside to get the kids. Stepping over the glass wall, now laying on the floor. The receptionist almost dropped, dead from shock. I had a hell of a headache for a day or so, or face ache, but never got a scratch. The next day my face wasn't even bruised!!

My life is full of disastrous vacations, and experiences, but I always laugh and love to tell my friends about them and make them laugh. They love to hear my stories.

Anyway at this particular time in my life, here I was, almost sixty years old, soon to be single again. Rejected by my handsome husband of sixteen years, and I didn't have a clue why!

I had to face selling my gorgeous new home, that I loved dearly. Starting my life all over at an age when I honestly thought I would be retiring.

That was the worst thing about a divorce at my age. After my first divorce it took me over two years, to trust someone again enough to consider getting into a second marriage. Even though things were not wonderful, I honestly believed we were headed in the same direction, and that we had the same mind in terms of retirement and what we would do with it. When my husband asked me for a divorce, it was the ultimate stab in the back, the ultimate betrayal. That thought was much more painful than the fact I was losing him. That the plans of sixteen years were all of a sudden invalid, and I had to start all over! That and the fact that I didn't have a clue what prompted it. He was not the sort of man to run around, he truly loved me, and thought I was beautiful even though I was a little over weight. To this day I really don't know why he did it, and I see him often. All he will say is we hadn't been getting along for a while. I believe it had to do with control. He was Sicilian, he had been a bachelor for fifty years, and he had become very neurotic since his cancer. Somewhere in that combination of things he decided he wanted control over his money his comings and goings and how he did things.

Here I was, a little over weight, doing a job that did not pay enough, had no money other than the house, no retirement, no benefits of my own, and low self esteem. It all seemed so overwhelming.

I've always been a survivor, and I've never been one to cry over spilled milk. The very next day "I picked myself up, brushed myself off and started all over again" as the song says. I decided to just face each day as it came. Thinking too far ahead would just scare me. I would put my best energies into the task at hand. Every day I would try to accomplish at least one thing toward my ultimate goal. Which at this time was to completely change my whole life!

My first twenty years I did not work. When I got my first divorce, I opened the coffee shop, and made a lot of money. I had stayed with restaurant work, after I had closed the shop, waitressing, bar tending, managing restaurants. That's all I had to put on my resume, which would just get me more restaurant jobs. Now, pushing sixty, I felt I had to make a change back toward the office work I had done as a teenager. We had come into the computer age and I was basically computer illiterate. I could not continue to carry heavy restaurant trays till I was seventy and beyond. I would love to take courses, but I had no extra time or money if I was working. I searched the papers every day for any type of office work. I made up a new resume, trying to play up the skills I had for managing, my work ethic, my good qualities rather than my experience. I got a few interviews, but to get a job in a bank or a store with no experience the most they would start you at was $8.00 an hour. In a restaurant with tips you made twice that, I could not afford to take such a cut and support myself. Finally, I came across a collection agency, that was willing to take me on at $9.00 an hour plus bonuses. They would train you on computers and other modern office equipment. They will usually hire anyone, even if you're half blind and seventy years old. The last thing in the world I wanted to do was collections, but if you can stick it out for just a couple of months, you will get the training you need to go on to something else. This was my thought when I took the job. Three months at most. There were many women working there in the same boat as I. Same age group and a lot of divorce situations. We became friends and supported one another not only at work but we began to socialize. Many were suffering from the same anxieties, and lack of self-esteem for the same reasons. They were between thirty-five and seventy, divorced or widowed and trying to support themselves and start over. The agency offered full benefits, and 401k that we could begin to start a retirement even at our advance ages. They matched some of it, which was great. The rest of the girls working there were twenty year old misfits, who couldn't afford to go to college, or were not smart enough, and were also trying to support themselves.

Within two months, I was the highest collector in the place and making at least a couple of hundred a month in bonuses. I was a natural for collections, I could empathize with the clients, and I would help them to figure out a budget that they could live with to pay their debt. A job I had intended to last two months, turned into years and I made great bonuses and got promoted several times. There are other jobs in collection agencies besides collections, you can do data processing, subrogation, insurance billing etc. They usually will not let you go for the other jobs, however until you've gotten your feet wet in collections. Don't be afraid to try it, they seldom ever fire anyone, they have too great a turnover and its easy to become a supervisor. No one wants to be one, but it looks great on your resume. I later went on to go to work for a hospital, where I am today.

When you first take a job like this, however, at your age. You are going to feel like the stupidest person in the world. Your going to ask your trainer the same questions a hundred times, but don't be afraid to ask them. Don't be afraid to admit out of the ten people she's training you're the only one who doesn't understand, because the others are lying. They trained ten of us at a time. Usually their were half older people and half twenty year olds. The older people couldn't see the computer screen, and you had to ask to sit in the front. The younger people would never ask a question and when the trainer would say do you understand that, they would always say yes, but they didn't as we found out when we actually started working. Us older ones who had driven the supervisor nuts asking questions, finally got it. The younger ones who said yes they understood everything didn't have a clue. So don't be afraid to say, no I don't understand, or can you show me that one more time. In the end when us old folks finally get it, it's there to stay!

*Change is a part of every life, resisting is often as futile as it is frustrating....*by Anonymous

I had started the collections job a short while before my husband had asked for the divorce, because I had been living on my own away from him part time for a while. For almost five years, I had been residing in the condo we had bought for our weekends in Portsmouth. He had been living in our house in Wolfeboro. It isn't as strange as it sounds, We lived apart because we owned both places, and our jobs necessitated it. We still got together on the weekends and it seemed fine.

We knew several couples our age that lived that way, and we actually thought at the time that it helped the marriage. We would not see each other all week, we would talk on the phone like a couple of teenagers, and on the weekend it would be like a honeymoon.

Now, I felt I was extremely grateful to have the job in collections, I figured I would stay there until I retired. When my husband asked for the divorce, I had to completely change my thought process and think in terms of how I was going to support myself for the rest of my life, I might never retire!

I had to access all avenues of financial possibility, as you need to. I had poured my heart, time and money into the house that was to be our retirement home. I had known from the minute I had walked in the door at that house, it was my house. I collected cobalt blue glass. The kitchen of this house had small cobalt blue ceramic tiles on all the counters. I loved an open concept house, with lofts, and cathedral ceilings, this house had all that. Our house in Wolfeboro and the condo in Portsmouth were also that style. The house was an older home that had been completely redone as a split-level. The kitchen and family room were upstairs, with a loft bedroom over the family room, a huge bath complete with hot tub, and a long deck off the family room completed the living quarters on the 2nd and 3rd floor. Down stair on the first level was a huge living room and master bedroom suite with a closed porch off the cathedral ceiling bedroom. It was absolutely gorgeous. We had sold the other two houses to buy it and it was paid in full. During the short time we owned it, I put a full length blue and crystal stained glass window in the family room, one we had designed ourselves at a cost of $3,000.00 and a crystal chandelier I had brought from Italy, it was aurora borealis and was hand made at the glass factory in Venice at a cost of over $1,000.00. I tell you this just so you will know, I had as much to give up as any of you. I had also recently purchased a rebuilt player piano, I just loved, and I had a fabulous collection of antique dolls worth over $35.000.00. All this with the intention of retiring there in comfort.

What I did and what you need to do, when you are by yourself, you have to look at this "stuff", not as treasured keep sakes, but as collateral. If you put it all together, how long can you live on what it will bring you. That may seem cold, but it's the truth. That's what I mean by looking at everything in a different way, and it's necessary to do this. Think of all that "stuff" as something I had, and I enjoyed for a time, but now its survival. When you are sixty years old and you are facing the rest of your life, you hang onto necessities and kiss everything else goodbye.

I did not know until I went to the Legal aid people that I was entitled to half of my husband's pension. This is an important thing that you must look into. I know that in Massachusetts and New Hampshire it's the law, I don't know about other states, but ask. This is not something that you have to worry about getting in court, its written in stone and its yours. Your husband cannot keep it from you, but you can negotiate it if you want. I believe it's for anyone married ten years or more, but again you can find out in your individual state what it is.

You do not need a lawyer for any of this just go to legal aid or to the family court, they will tell you what to do and give you the paper work you need. You are also, if you are married a certain amount of time, entitled to half of your husbands social security. This is a piddely amount however and you might prefer to work on your own. If you have always worked, no sweat, but if your like me and didn't for a lot of years, or worked for yourself you are going to have to start working now to get your right amount when you retire.

If your husband dies, you are entitled to widow's benefits, even if you are divorced. You want to look into all these things and don't listen to one word your husband says on it. My husband went nuts when he found out I was entitled to half of his pension, I am sure that was one of the factors in his asking for the divorce anyway, and when he found out he was not going to be in total control of it he went nuts.

This made it easier for me to negotiate, You can offer him to buy back your share of the pension if you wish. It depends on the amount and what the deal is on his pension if he dies. Would you be the beneficiary or would he be able to leave it to someone else. In my case I figured out how much it would be worth over say twenty years, and I offered to let him buy it from me for $40,000.00 I convinced him it would be a good deal. Then I invested the money in blue chip stocks with a financial advisor.

I picked aggressive stocks to make it grow faster. They invest it in such a way you won't ever lose it, it may go up and down but when one thing goes down the other goes up. It's very diversified. I also wanted to be done with him and any connections. Now its my money and I can do what I want with it. He was thrilled to be able to keep all his money. I also got half the money from the house when it was sold. I used that to buy a small condo, I could afford. I paid cash for it so my expenses for living are just the taxes and condo fees.

You want to come away with the best deal and the most money you can. You need to invest, to make your own little nest egg for your future. Of course you can opt to take half the pension in monthly installments, but be sure if he dies the pension doesn't die with him or you could wind up with nothing.

I also bought from him at the time, two pieces of property that we had in Vegas. He had always thought it was a waste of our money and wanted to be done with it. We had bought them over ten years ago, for $18,000.00 for both pieces. It was land that was not being built on yet, he let me have them after some negotiation for $2,000.00. I have already sold one for $7,000.00 and invested that money and still have the other one. You have to be clear headed despite your state of mind. If you are not and he is, you will find yourself getting taken and wondering later how you got in this state.

Do not take his first offer on anything, act disinterested. For instance the first time my ex offered me the land, he wanted $10,000.00 for it. I just laughed and said what do I want that for? No, I'm not interested. Later he came back with the $2,000.00 and I reluctantly agreed.

I believe in being fair, but he is much more capable than you of continuing to make money. With some exceptions. Never make financial decisions in the heat of passion. When you are alone, sit down and put down on paper everything you own together, don't forget a thing. Then come up with an equitable way of dividing it. In our case when it came to the contents of the house, we decided just to take a day, go into each room and pick. He could have first pick and then me , back and forth until everything was gone. Put it all down on paper, two lists, his side and yours. When everything is gone, both of you sign the paper and make three copies, one for you, one for him and one to be held by a third non involved party. That way when you start moving stuff out, if any of your stuff disappears you will know it and have proof its yours.

Be smart about what you take, when you do your division. Think about it for a few days before. Take things you need for your new home, or things you can turn into money.

My ex was thinking only of taking things, he thought would hurt me or things he thought he could sell, but was unaware of how much they would really bring.

The day we sorted our stuff it went something like this. He picked things he thought I wanted the most. He had first pick, he chose our 53-inch television set, I took the player piano. He took the Venetian chandelier, I took the living room sectional, He took my cobalt blue chandelier, and I took the dining room table and chairs. So when we were done, I had enough to furnish my apartment. He had an assortment of blue glassware, a television too big for most apartments, a bunch of animal figurines, he barely took a bed or chair. He sold most of what he took for dirt, I think he got a couple of hundred dollars for the television that had cost us over $2,000.00 and in the end, he couldn't sell the chandeliers and he wound up selling them back to me. He later regretted his choices when he tried to furnish a place. I have only half the cobalt I used to have, and a mish mosh of furniture but my place looks great, very eclectic or bohemian. I sent my doll collection to auction, it broke my heart, but I didn't have room in a small place for 200 dolls. I got a fraction of the worth, but I invested it and didn't look back.

You have to adopt a "less is more" theory. You need only the basics, you will always have your memories. Now its time to start making new memories, you don't need the old to sustain you. Think of it this way, only old people surround themselves with a bunch of old stuff. Young people never do. You are a new "young" person, new life , new to the world. Let your new place reflect this new life. It's also expensive to store "stuff" you are not going to use again. Don't think about, I might need this some day. If you do, you can buy a new one with the money you save on storage, and chances are you will never need it again, if you don't need it now. New life, new thought process!

I promise you, once you are in that little pad, and you own it outright. You will feel so good, to know it's yours and no one can take it away from you. You can afford it, you won't be stressed wondering where you are going to go and how you're going to survive. I look around now at my place and I can't even remember what I had before.

I have a very dear girlfriend. She has been divorced longer than I have. She had her own business, and a beautiful home. Her husband ran off with her secretary leaving her in her late fifties to face life alone, she was devastated. She is a gorgeous, beautiful woman, she has the most beautiful face. She still years later cannot get a grip. She has not moved on with her life. She is working at the collection agency, but she is very reluctant to take a promotion or to rock the boat. She is far more intelligent than I am, but she cannot seem to regain her self-confidence. She has gained a lot of weight, she is in a job she hates, and she is in a rented apartment. She has all her "stuff" stored. She keeps bringing home boxes from the storage and going through all that "stuff" from her past. Her apartment is littered with all this "stuff" she can't get rid of, Get rid of it!!

So, to reiterate, at the time of my divorce, I had been working at the collection agency for a couple of years. I was doing well there, and intended to stay till I retired, because unlike a lot of people working there I liked it. I had no idea that there was any way a person, my age could get a better job, or make more money. I kept my eye on the bulletin board at work and any time a promotion would be offered that was up my alley, I would apply. I had no desire to be a supervisor, to me they were just glorified baby sitters and I didn't want to deal with that. I know at our age any change is scary but you know what you are capable of doing. In our company, they will let you try a new job and if you don't feel its what you like after a couple of weeks they will let you return to the old job. Ask about that, if you see an offer posted. Or ask ahead of time about working with someone as a trainee in a position you think you would like, while doing your own job. I did that a couple of times, before actually taking a new position. I applied for a job as an assistant to the boss. It was something different, but after a couple of weeks, I realized it was too boring for me and I told her. They put me back into my old position, no problem and I had in the couple of weeks learned a few new things, that I could add to my resume.

I tried a couple of different positions, until they promoted me to "customer service rep". I would be on the road, visiting clients, a dream job for me. This happened within the first year of my divorce, and I thought things were really going well for me. Unfortunately, it caused a supervisor in the company, who had been my boss and whom I had gotten along very well with for five years, to turn on me. She didn't like the man who was my new boss, and didn't like the fact that I had been promoted out of her department. She began using all her influence to have me demoted back into her department. She was so adamant in her desire to do it, she even lied and put things into my personal file, which up to now had been exemplary.

She was eventually found out, but not before she had succeeded in having me demoted back to my old position.

At first I had been extremely hurt, but being in my financial position, I felt helpless to do anything about it. After some thought on it, and my hurt changing to anger, I decided they were not going to get away with it. I had always loved the company, but they had not stood by me, and needed a lesson. A new company was opening up in town, doing medical collections, I went to see the new managers. I not only succeeded in negotiating a great package for myself, but I took eighteen of the best people from the old company with me. I personally got a decent raise and was allowed to work a four-day week, which I had always wanted to do. It dealt a deadly blow to the old company, they lost one of their biggest clients. For a few months, we enjoyed the new company, we knew everyone in the office and it was a much friendlier atmosphere than the old one. After about six months, however this company was bought out by a new company with much more strict ways of conducting their business, we all became, unhappy . I was beginning to be discouraged, but so far every move had been a positive one so again out went the resumes. I had two great interviews, the first company wanted me badly, but it was no advantage over what I had. The second one was at the local hospital and they gave me still another raise and a much easier job following up on Insurance companies .

These experiences showed me no matter what your age, or fears, with enough determination and grit, you can and will succeed at what ever you choose. I found that a good interview far outweighs the best resume, if they like your personality, if you have good work ethic, if your not late or have a lot of absences your in. I found out after the fact, that quite a few girls had applied for the job I got. Some much younger and smarter. The hospital is very particular and the average job interview goes like this. You apply, two female supervisors interview you. If they like you, they pass word on to a male supervisor over the entire office Mark. He will hear their opinion and call you in for an interview. If he like you he will pass word on to Human resources who will take an complete job application that will have to pass a security check, extensive background check, and then you will be tested for several diseases etc. If that is all o.k. you will be hired. A little scary for anyone, but especially us old broads who are already overly self-conscious, and self-critical anyway. Also, I must tell you, I seldom dress in a business conservative way. For a job interview, I may wear a business suit but I try to alter it to my style so they won't be surprised later. I am not saying you should not dress in a business manner, you should, but I want them to know up front I am an individual.

I went for my first interview with the two ladies, early on a Friday morning my day off. I gave them a list of my strengths right off, and tried to be very relaxed and self-assured. I kidded around a little, and also told them what I considered to be my weaknesses. At the end of the interview, they asked if I could stay around a while and see if Mark was in the building so he could interview me right away. I said sure, Mark was there and he interviewed me immediately. I was the same with him, relaxed, personable, played up my strengths. I also however, tried to get him to give me the four-day week I was now working, and told him about two vacations I already had planned. He countered by telling me the vacations were fine, he could not give me the four-day week, but could give me a decent raise. I hedged a little, he asked when I could start. By the time I got home, two miles away the Human resources dept called and wanted me to come right over for the testing and to make out the applications for back ground checks, Mark had hand carried my resume over there. I started working on Monday! I tell you this because, I half bluffed my way through the interview. I was nervous I was very unsure of myself, but I didn't let it show. I still had the other job, if I didn't get it, I didn't get it. But, I did! Some of my girlfriends who are still at the original company, envy me and would like to do the same, but they are too afraid. They are worried about their security, which is a true worry, but you are not going to advance without some risk. You cannot be reckless, but you have to develop initiative, and be aggressive.

You win or loose it at the interview, plan it in you head ahead of time. Be yourself, try to smile and laugh, look them straight in the eye, keep your head up. Brag about your strengths. If there is something in the job description you know you might need training in, tell them right then, but follow up with I will give it my best. I am a fast learner. Don't be afraid to tell them something personal, about yourself that will show your initiative.

Companies like people with a good work ethic, good attendance, neat dresser, good sense of humor and self-starter.

Life is either a daring adventure, or nothing! Helen Keller

Chapter eight:

The Dating Game! Can I face this again!

If you don't like it change it, If you don't want to change it, it can't be that bad! ....Anonymous

    I guess the scariest part, of beginning to go again is. Will anyone like me? Am I too old for this scene? Would anyone ever find me attractive? Do I have the energy for it? Can I find any women in my situation to go out with me? and in my case, will I be able to drive myself around at night, with the problem I have seeing after dark.?
    I had faced all these same problems , when I was divorced at forty-three, but now they were highly escalated, giving twenty more years.
    I found the girlfriends, right at work, there were many, many who were dying to get out, but just kept talking about it. They needed an organizer who would plan it and tell them you be ready Saturday night and I'll pick you up ! Of course there are also, a lot who won't go out. They will tell you how lonely, and depressed they are, but when you offer a solution, its "I wouldn't be caught dead in a singles bar!" Of course they have never been in one, but they have a definite opinion of what one is. The average singles, is not a bar. It more closely resembles a club, sort of like an elks club or moose hall, except they are always populated by just men. The set up is similar, a big hall, with either a bar you can set at or maybe just a service bar. A big dance floor, a buffet table, and a lot of smaller tables holding two to ten people. It usually costs about $5.00 to get in, their is a dress code, and you get a hot buffet and an evening of socializing and dancing

and drinking or not depending on your preference. Men love it because its reasonably priced, they get a hot meal without cooking and theirs lots of other guys to hide behind while they are looking for a woman. The women love it, because they get to dress up, socialize with their friends, dance, look over the assortment of men, and make fun of them with the other girls.

It's really quite fun, and even if its not your scene you need to go at least once or twice, so when your talking about it in the future you can talk with some intelligence, instead of just sounding like a sour old maid.

I love to dress up and I like my men dressed up, and its one of the few places you can go to do that. At my age I do not want to go out with a guy with his baseball hat turned around back wards on his head and it stays on right through dinner.

So, as I mentioned earlier in this book, my first few times I went out was with a group of five to eight girls, that just sort of migrated to each other, our first nights out were just going downtown to a jazz club and sitting and getting to know each other and the musicians. We learned to enjoy the music, the musicians and the arty, eccentric people who hung out there. They were interesting and different and I loved it. You begin to realize that while you were living your careful little married life, there was a whole world going on you never experienced, and it gives new excitement to this new single state you are in. After a few weeks, the sameness got a little boring, I can listen to good music only so long without dancing, so when and older couple we know, suggested we go dancing at the Ashworth, we jumped at the chance. The Ashworth is a hotel at Hampton beach, and it has a great disc jockey every night.

The first time we went over, there were about eight girls and one guy. The one guy, belonged to the oldest of us girls, and they had just met, a few months before and were very much in love. It was cute to see a couple in their late sixties in love like a couple of teenagers. He was a lot of fun and enjoyed dancing. We were all sitting around one table, watching the guys coming in hoping someone would ask us to dance. I spotted two Italian looking guys come in the door. One was tall and fairly handsome, dark curly hair. The other was shorter, interesting looking but not handsome, kind of looked like Gregory Hines the dancer. As I watched them, trying to get the tall ones attention, the shorter one spotted me. Much to my dismay, he asked me to dance. I was happy to dance so I accepted, he turned out to be a hot shit. Great personality, and very attentive. His name was Sam, and he was adorable. He had recently moved here from Florida, was retired, was in the middle of a divorce from a much younger woman in Florida. He was very leery of becoming involved, but was attracted to me enough to ask for my number. Not bad first time out and a guy asks for my number.

At that time, I was living out of my car on the weekends, or at my sisters. My ex was still coming to Portsmouth on the weekend, and we hadn't sold the house yet. Until we did, unless I wanted to spend the weekend with him, which I didn't I got out every Friday after work and didn't go back till Sunday night. So when I went to work on Friday morning I packed the car for the weekend.

By the way, I did get to dance with the tall one that night, but he turned out to be a real jerk, that's something you learn quickly, the attractive ones are not always the best ones. Too bad guys don't learn that about women, as Judge Judy says, "Beauty fades dumb is forever!"

That Sunday, as I was hanging around my sister's house, trying to think of something to do, that wouldn't cost money, the phone rang. It was Sam, he said he was cooking and would love to invite me for dinner. He lived fairly close by my sisters, so I accepted and rode over there.

He had a third floor apartment, inexpensive but cute with a little schnauzer dog. The only problem I was very allergic to dogs and cats. I also found out Sam smoked like a chimney and that reacted on my allergies too. That afternoon, after some excellent homemade wine and spaghetti dinner, we took a ride to Lawrence. It was either that or I would have sneezed all day.

We went to a little neighborhood bar that belonged to a friend of his. It was an Italian and Irish bar. It was the first time I had ever heard of those two races in the same breath, but here it was all very compatible. They were having a Pre super bowl party, it was sometime in December. There was a good representation of both Irish and Italians there and I got to know them all. They were all very attentive, and made me feel fantastic. I had an Irish cop on one side, and an Italian on the other and they were both telling me they were much better catches than Sam. The Irish cop told me he had never seen anyone, more strikingly beautiful! Even if he was full of shit, no one had ever called me strikingly beautiful. I wanted to stay there forever!

We had a lot of laughs and a great time. At the end of the afternoon, Sam announced we had to go home and stir the spaghetti. They all yelled, you go home and stir the spaghetti, leave her with us! Sam and I began to see each other on a regular basis after that, but I continued to go out with the girls. I wasn't ready to jump into a relationship and neither was he. Besides if I was he wasn't really what I wanted, he was just good company for the time being. The girls and I started going to a singles dance in Nashua, on Fridays and Saturday nights. At the beginning I hooked a ride with them, I was still not able to drive after dark. I could make it from work to Sam's, about four or five miles and that was it.

The first Saturday night I went with them, I just wore slacks, a sweater and fashion boots, it was cold and winter and I didn't think. I had remembered from when I was single at forty, that the guys always stand in groups, either where the food is or at the bar. So I stood by the buffet table part of the time. The girls, got a table, but a table of six or eight girls is very intimidating for a guy to approach. I got asked to dance a couple of times, but I noticed the girls who were getting asked the most, were wearing short dresses and high heels.

So the following week, I wore a short swingy dress, and high heels, I didn't sit down all night. I have great legs and they noticed! I never went out without meeting at least two new guys, the girls began to be a little jealous, they had been going a lot longer than I had and one or two of them had met guys but three or four of them didn't dance all night and of course got discouraged. I knew what they were doing wrong, but it was hard to tell them. I went out to eat, with a few guys I met, but I still didn't have my own place, and I wasn't going to travel to Nashua, (maybe fifty miles), so at first that was the extent of my dating. I was still seeing Sam, and I spent a couple of nights a week at his house. He would cook me dinner after work, he would read the paper and get involved in the television set, something I was not interested in. I would go to bed early, he would stay up all night, I had to go to work, he could sleep till noon.

The more I saw him the more I knew he was not the one for me. We had become good friends, he was good to talk to and I could spend the weekend there if I wanted to. He got jealous if I went out with someone else but he wasn't willing to take me out, or give up the smoking or anything else to help our relationship. He loved going out with his "Goombas", he was a sweet man, he adored me, but not on a permanent basis. He would cook for me, drive me around, go with me to jazz with the girls on Sunday nights, because he loved jazz.

The payoff was, one night I was getting ready to leave work, it had been snowing all afternoon and it had really piled up. Sam's house was maybe four miles up the road, mine was eight or nine miles down the road. I called him to see if I could come over and stay. First he said sure, but he called me back and said no I couldn't because he was going to a bar in Boston with a friend of his. I said have you looked outside its terrible, you should not be on the road! On top of that, I knew when he went out with his friends they always got smashed, I could not imagine them driving to Boston and back in that terrible storm drunk. He would not change his mind, he said I was worrying too much he was going. I was not only mad that he would venture out on such a night but that he was not even thinking of me getting home safe! I was very upset with him and that was the beginning of the end.

I started going to a dance on Sunday night in Salem N.H.. I usually went to that one with just one of the girls I went out with on Friday and Saturday. The others, just could not go out two or three nights in a row. I could go out every night given the chance. Beverly and I went to Salem every week for a while.

The very first time we went, there was a young guy who came over to ask me to dance. He was fairly attractive, a little overweight, but beautiful blue eyes and a very gentle face. I danced with him a couple of times, I found out he was twenty years younger than me, so when he kept asking me and getting more attentive, I told him no, ask someone your own age. I told him I was not interested in a man young enough to be my son. He was not discouraged, he kept asking. Finally, I thought oh well what the hell, we're just dancing. So I said to him in jest, ok, I'll dance with you, but I'm not having your babies, besides I had the baby factory taken out and a playground put in. He thought that was the funniest thing he ever heard. He laughed and laughed. Bev was not meeting anyone, and she wanted to go home so we left. Somehow, he got my number, I don't know how. He started calling every night asking me out.

I always refused him, but he never got discouraged, he kept telling me the age thing didn't matter. Some nights he would call a couple of times, but I still refused to go out with him.

Then suddenly it was almost New Years Eve, one of my favorite nights out. I asked Sam if he wanted to go out. He said he hated to go out on New Years Eve. I asked him if he wanted me to get a bottle of champagne, and we could go out for a quiet supper and then have champagne at his house. He said he didn't want to make plans.

That night Mike, the young guy called, asked me what I was doing for New Years, I was mad at Sam, so I said not a dam thing. He asked me if I wanted to go out for dinner and dancing and I jumped at the chance.

We went out that night and had a wonderful time. We went for a prime rib dinner and then to a club for dancing. He was a perfect gentleman, and great company. He was extremely attentive, and renewed feelings in me I hadn't experienced for a while. I had intended to go home, but I stayed over at his house.

After that we began going out on a regular basis, we always had a great time. He was extremely attentive, money was no object, and he always bought me roses, . We went out to Comedy clubs, dining , dancing anything I wanted to do. He showered me with gifts. When

I remarked on the way he dressed, he went out and bought a whole new wardrobe, letting me help pick it out. I found one of the reasons, I didn't like going out with a younger man is the way they dress. The younger generation thinks dressed up is jeans, a baseball jacket or one with some logo on it, baseball caps, and always sneakers. Mike had worn a suit on New Years and he looked terrific, but the rest of the time, he dressed as I have just described. I explained this to him and he completely changed. He bought several sport coats, he wore even with his jeans, he bought more dress shoes, shirts and ties, and suits. He always dressed when he went out with me. I continued going out with the girls, but I saw Mike at least two nights a week. I continued to protest the age difference, but it didn't matter to him. The sex was fantastic, he kept telling me it was the best he had ever had, he said no one his age was ever able to keep up with him. He never got tired, he could keep going all night one time right after another.

The more men I dated closer to my age, the more disappointed I became in them. Mike kept looking better and better. I would say at least one in three men over the age of fifty-five, cannot perform sexually without Viagra.

Many of them have high blood pressure, and the medication they take makes them unable to sustain an erection. They will come on strong and then nothing, they would be better off, not to come on strong in the first place. They also have not gotten the message that alcohol keeps most men from performing. They all drink too much. It wasn't just the sexual performance, however, it was their general lack of energy. If they go out two nights a week they are wiped. I have an excessive amount of energy for my age, I cannot be a couch potato, its just not possible. Also most men do not like to dance. They go to the singles to pick someone up, or meet someone, they dance because they have to . After they meet you they expect to be able to stop dancing. Not with me , dancing is my favorite thing to do.

Most of the men over fifty five or sixty their lives are, watching sports on TV, hanging out at their local coffee shop or club, and reading the paper. If they have any extra energy they play golf with the guys.

As Mike and I became closer, he began to get jealous of my going out with the girls, so against my better judgment, I stopped, and went out with him exclusively. Then after a couple of months, my house had still not been sold, he suggested I move in with him until I got settled. It seemed like a good idea at the time. He had a nice big house, I was still living in my car on the weekend, and because the house was still not sold and everyone was loosing their patience the divorce was starting to get a little bitter. Mostly because my husband didn't want to give me his pay check any more, but he expected me to keep paying the household bills. There was no way, we could pay household bills and support two single life styles as well.

Mikes suggestion would settle the problem for now. He helped me move just my clothes, My music, and my exercise equipment in his house. I told Mike it was strictly on a trial basis, he agreed. If either of us didn't like it I would move back out. He was so elated that I was moving in, he would agree to anything.

I tried to make a normal life for us. He had terrible eating habits, he would starve all day and then order Chinese or Pizza. As much as I loved Chinese or Pizza, I knew that could not be a normal daily eating pattern and I could see why he was over weight. I shopped and cooked healthy and delicious meals for us every night. He would remark how good it was but seldom eat a whole meal. He would say I'll eat it later. I did his laundry and fixed up the house. He had nice furniture, but the curtains were in rags, from the person who owned it before him. He had no pictures, or bedspreads or any decorations. I decorated the house beautifully, he loved it. He gave me any money I needed for the house or food. Sometimes, if he was going to be working in the yard all day he would give me money and send me to the mall to shop for myself.

Everything seemed to be going ok I took a trip to Spain with friends, a few weeks after we were living together, we missed each other terribly. I had planned the trip way before I had any knowledge of the possibility of divorce. I needed the trip and it was paid for. I needed to get away with my girlfriends and look at things with a clear head. Spain was magnificent, the architecture, was like something out of the Arabian nights. We had a wonderful time in the evenings walking around Madrid, and Barcelona. The weather was grand. I had a great time, but I missed Mike, we called each other every day.

I had to cut my trip short because of an abscessed tooth. They had tried to treat it at a hospital in Spain, but it just made it worse. They put me on an antibiotic that caused me to swell, my eyes my cheeks, I had to come home. Never go on a long trip, without buying the insurance. They made arrangements for me to come home alone. From a small town in Spain, to a major airport to pickup my ticket. No one spoke English. I looked like a deformed freak.

Mike waited at the airport almost twenty four hours for my plane to get in. He must really love me to do that. He was so worried. I was so happy to see him, we really missed each other. Little did I know however, there was a devil lurking in our home, I was unaware of. One Saturday it finally reared its ugly head. We had made plans to go out for dinner and dancing that evening. He was going to spend the day working in the yard. I was cleaning and doing laundry. Every once in while he would come in to give me a kiss, and see if everything was alright. I would assure him it was. He offered to give me money to go shopping I told him I was fine and looking forward to our evening. About five he came in to get cleaned up. I was all ready way ahead of him, as I always was, and prodding him to hurry up.

He was a slow mover, always, and if we had reservations at seven he would still be getting ready at seven. This was one of those nights. We were in the bedroom, I noticed he had done his shirt up wrong, I reached over to help him, kidding him about it being wrong. When I did he pulled away from me, and fell over on the bed. When he hit the bed he was unconscious. Like in a deep sleep, I shook him and could not wake him. Then I realized he was dead drunk. I couldn't figure out how he could get drunk so fast. He had seemed o.k. all day. He must have been drinking all day to get that drunk he would be unconscious. I was so upset I left him that way half dressed, left the light on and went downstairs to sleep. I was extremely disappointed at not going out. I fell asleep on the couch, I woke up about three in the morning and went upstairs to check on him. He was still laying exactly as I had left him, light still on, still dressed. I left him again and went back down stairs. About five in the morning I was awakened by some one gently shaking me. Sweetheart, what are you doing down here? I looked up, he was in a robe standing over me. I sat up. Don't you remember what happened ? He didn't, we talked about it, I told him I came from a family of alcoholics I would not deal with one. If he had a problem I would move out. He assured me he did not and it would never happen again.

I had a great deal of experience with alcoholics, besides my grandfather, my mother who disappeared when I was sixteen, my baby sisters husband had been one. He was the perfect father for sixteen years, never drinking except on New Years eve when he would get dead drunk. Then he would not drink till the next New Years eve. Every New Years eve he would drink until he passed out, but that was the only time he did it. Then after being the perfect husband and father for sixteen years, he lost his job. When it went into a few months he started drinking, he became a wife beater, he could not take the kidding from his brothers and other people that his wife was the breadwinner all of a sudden. My sister would turn up on my porch beat to a pulp. I would go down his house and scream at him and go after him. Eventually a man he picked on in a bar murdered him. It was such a wasted life, he was such a great guy when he didn't drink. I despised alcohol and would not put up with someone who abused it.

During the next few weeks, I was cleaning out a lot of old drawers at his suggestion, when I came across some paper work from a couple of years before. Mike had been arrested for drunk driving and had gone to AA. I brought it up to him and he gave me hell for snooping. I told him he had told me to clean out the drawers I was not snooping, he finally admitted he had a problem but assured me it was behind him. I started watching him more closely.

A couple of weeks later, the same thing happened, he had been working in the yard all day, we were planning to go out to dinner and dancing. I had been watching him closely and had seen nothing. I saw no bottle except maybe one bottle of beer he had with a neighbor who had wandered into the yard. We were getting ready to go out, he came in from the shower and dropped unconscious on the bed. I was furious, but this time I was not staying in and confronting him, I would go out by myself. I got dressed and left. I had no idea where I was going to go. I had heard of a singles in Danvers Ma. but I had never been there. I had no idea how to get there from Salem. It was raining and I looked like shit. Up till that night I had not driven in the dark, the rain made the reflections even worse, I didn't care I just wanted to get away. I was so mad, I was determined to go somewhere, I drove up and down the high way for a while trying to decide should I go to the Ashworth or try to find the place in Danvers.? I opted for Danvers and went there alone. I wound up having a fantastic time, everyone asked me to dance. I went in alone and knew no one, but by the time I left I knew a lot of people. After the dance I drove back to my sisters, she had given me a key and I let myself in and went to bed. In the morning I talked to her about it, she could relate, she was the one who's husband was an alcoholic and had been murdered years before. I made up my mind I was moving out of Mikes.

    I called my oldest son, and told him, he came down and helped me move my stuff out. Mike was very upset, but I told him I would not be with a drunk, I could not see him any more. My son was very kind to him, but got all my
stuff for me.

My ex was not happy to see me move back in the house.

We decided we needed to get a new real estate person, our house had been on the market more than six months and was getting no movement.

    I got together with four or five recommended agents, had them all come to the house and talk to me about it. I went with the one that was the most excited about it, he raised the price, put it on the computer and sold it in three days. Don't ever be afraid to do something new, different and unexpected. My old realtor told me the house was overpriced! He had been a great help in the selling of my condo before, but on this house he was just not the right one. It was still another month, of packing and sorting and moving etc. but finally that particular chapter was closed. I moved into my own little condo, which I purchased outright with my half of the house money. Finally I felt independent again, it was a real relief to close that door, and get on with my life. My ex had tried a couple of little deals at the end to wind up with more money than he was supposed to, but I cut him off at the pass each time. For instance, we had a lot of credit card debt that was supposed to come off the top of the sale. The company that writes the checks for the house, will only write so many checks. They will pay off your old mortgage, they will divide the money in two but they won't write individual checks for your bills. That money has to go into one of your checks, either you or your ex. You have to be sure that whichever one gets it will pay those bills. My ex wanted it in his check, I knew that was to my advantage, because when you have to pay taxes later, its better for you if your check is less. So I agreed, but now I had to be sure he paid off the bills. I had made the deal with him to buy back the chandeliers I loved. He had brought them to the closing and put them in my car. After the checks were distributed I wanted him to write out checks for the credit cards in my presence. He refused to do that. So I just took off, without giving him the money for the chandeliers. He called me about it and I told him when I saw the checks for the bills I would give him that $1,000.00 not until. He was mad but he wrote them.

No more house bills, the divorce was final, things were looking up. I settled into my little home, and was happier than I had been in years.

Unfortunately, I was not done with Mike though. An Odyssey began that lasted another two years. He would call me crying, promising to stay off the booze. He would go on a binge of not eating, he would exercise, buy great looking new clothes, look good for a while, and then fall off the wagon with one greater spill than the one before. He would try to bribe me with gifts, offer to take me to plays or places he knew I wanted to go. If I had a problem with my car, he would offer to fix it. I would give in, give him another chance, and he would always blow it by getting drunk. He was forever getting himself hurt, because he was doing things drunk half the time.

One time that he was working on my car, he opened the radiator while it was hot and burned his face all up. Anyone knows you can't do that. Another time he ran into a tree while skiing, A truck hit him in the head with its mirror while he was jogging. It was just one thing after another. Each time I would swear off seeing him forever, but he would call me five times a day, vowing all kinds of things if I would just give him another chance and he would wear me down. He offered me homes, and told me if I would marry him I would never have to work again, anything to get me to come back.

Every single week he sent a dozen long stem peach roses to my work. He took me to Boston and offered to buy me diamond rings, I kept telling him all I wanted was for him to give up the booze and live a normal life. He joined AA he went to the meetings and would come home and drink. He lied to me about it all the time.

Finally the inevitable happened he lost his license from drunk driving. He was extremely upset, worried about how he was going to get back and forth from work. He had just bought a brand new suburban vehicle. He made arrangements at first to have someone pick him up, but eventually he drove himself, without a license. He kept my life in a turmoil, because he was always calling. I would go out on a date and come home and there would be five or six messages from him. He always wanted to know where the girls and I were going, but I would never tell him. Sometimes, he would figure it out and show up drunk, and embarrass me, but even drunk, if I told him to leave he would.

He went more and more down hill. He constantly called and made promises, it was on the verge of stalking. Several times I gave in and went over his house to find him out cold on the bed with a bottle of VO by his bed. I tried to be a "friend" for a while, I offered to go over on Saturday and take him grocery shopping etc. since he was not supposed to be driving. Sometimes, I would find him good, and then it would be the old Mike and we would really talk. He would tell me how much he loved me and how he would do anything for me. I would tell him, I wanted only one thing, for him to get well, healthy and off the booze and make a good life for himself.

He would promise but it wouldn't last. I noticed that even when he didn't drink for a few days, it had taken its toll, he would shake and stagger. I begged him to go to a doctor for a check up. He finally did and they told him his blood pressure was sky high and put him on medication. When he was drinking he would forget to take it. One day he fell at work and split his head open. They lugged him off to the Hospital, they discovered he had a seizure. Now they put him on seizure medicine as well, but he was told he could not drink and take that medicine. He kept all this from his only relatives, his mother and two sisters. If he was invited to a family function he just would not go, or he would drive himself. He was stopped again and this time, was under threat to go to jail for driving without a license. As he went down hill the calls to me became more and more frequent. Even when I started going steady with another man, he would still call and talk to him.

He eventually lost his job, we begged him to get help, his lawyer kept getting a postponement on the charges. He was scared to death of going to jail but still would not check himself in for rehab. Finally this year on Holy Saturday just before Easter, we got a call from his neighbor. They found him dead in his house. Forty years old and he had killed himself, from neglect and booze. The coroner said it was a heart attack, but I know it was induced from not taking his medications, and drinking water glasses of VO with a Budweiser chaser. We felt terrible but had done all we could. He was a wonderful and gentle man when he was not drinking. I loved him very much at one time, and gave him every chance I could. I talked to his mother and sisters at his wake, they secretly suspected he was having problems but had no idea what. This whole thing took a good two years to go down, and during that time, I was living my life and having a good time. It was interspersed with these incidents scattered through out, my life at the time.

The first summer I was in my condo on my own, was the most exhilarating of my life. I became the most popular woman on the

North shore dating circuit. No one was more surprised with my popularity than I. Every time I went out with a new man, I could do no wrong. I was thinner, than I had ever been, I was in a size eight. I had my hair done, and artificial nails. I went dancing at the singles, either alone or with the girls, every Saturday, Sunday, Tuesday and Friday nights.

At one time, I was dating seven or eight men at a time. I went out to dinner almost every night in the week, they were all professional, attractive, interesting men. They took me to the best restaurants. I went every where. I never wanted it to change, I was constantly complimented, fawned over, my life was perfect. The women at the singles envied me and wanted to hang around me. Everyone was my friend. I could not believe it myself, I could not figure out why they were having such a hard time.

It was strictly in the way, I handled myself, as I have outlined in other chapters in this book. They couldn't seem to get it, but to me it came natural. I was by nature independent, and had no desire to change it, I didn't want to "hook" any guy for permanent. I let them know that and that attracted them to me like bees to honey. I was in awe of the attention I received and every single time I went out another, and another would want my phone number. I was very particular however, and I would not give it out to just anybody. During the time I had seven of them on the string, I had no room for any more, and I would tell them that. Consequently the men I went out with were really special, as far as I could tell at the time.

One of the first, was Jon. I met Jon, late one night at Hampton Beach. He was tall, handsome, and had the most beautiful blue eyes I had ever seen. A little cookie duster moustache. He looked like Errol Flynn. I was at the Ashworth, it was the end of the evening. I had a great time and was thinking about going home. He sat down near me at the bar, I said Hi, introduced myself and we started to talk. He was well tanned, and gorgeous. We talked till they threw us out. He lived nearby so I gave him a ride home. He invited me in for a cup of tea. I went in and we just talked some more.

He had lost his wife to cancer a year before. They had been

married thirty-seven years. At first he thought, I was too young for him, but when he found out I was older than him he was tickled. He was in his middle fifties. What was bizarre about the whole thing was. He had promised his three daughters, that he would not have anything to do with another woman for at least a year. During his marriage he had never been with another woman, and he had kept his vow for the past year. When I met him, he had another two weeks to go. I thought it was a bit much but I told him I respected his wishes and thought it was a nice gesture. I could tell he was smitten with me right away, and was wishing he did not have this hanging over his head. We said our goodnights and I went home. Next morning bright and early, he called and invited my girl friend and me to breakfast. We were going down town to a fair, so we invited him along. My girl friend thought he was gorgeous also. He walked us all over the fair, bought us roses, and food, and we talked a lot more. I discovered his daughters pretty much regulated his life.

Their intentions were good, and honorable, but it was the worst thing they could have done to help their father. By making him take an oath, that he would not have anything to do with another woman for at least a year after their mother's death. All that was left to him, was to drink and work to try to forget everything else. Instead of facing things and getting on with his life normally. It's normal and natural to seek out companionship, to talk to and let your emotions and feelings out. Every time a woman came up to him and started a conversation and he began to feel warm toward her, he would think of his oath and excuse himself. It didn't work with me, I encouraged him to tell me all about it, and to ask him how he felt about it, and to assure him he was not a bad person or an unfaithful husband because he wanted a relationship. Too much damage had been done over the year, however, he had become dependent on liquor, he slept too much, smoked too much, and let his daughters make his decisions.

During the next two weeks, we talked a lot. I tried to undo the damage they had done. He slept over my house a couple of times, but we did not have sex or anything. He would drink and smoke until he fell asleep, then it was almost impossible to wake him for work.

After a couple of times, and I saw what his habits were, I told him he couldn't stay over any more. I had enough trouble with Mike and his drinking problems, I didn't need another one. I felt very sorry for Jon though and knew he needed help and companionship. I encouraged him to come by the club on Saturday night and dance and call. He often left me bouquets of flowers on my car, or in my door. I would find them on my way to work. When the year was over, and he was "allowed" to have sex again, he still was not able to do it. He had denied himself too long and the guilt had become a part of him. That made him even more depressed, and he drank more.

He would often call or send a card, and take me out to breakfast. Sometimes he would come by the club at 10:30pm or later and have a few last dances with me. He was extremely complimentary and he told me several times, how much he cared for me and if he could have a relationship with anyone he wanted it to be me. We would sometimes kiss and make out to a point, but he just could not let himself go beyond that. I did all I could for him, it was such a waste. He was sweet, attentive, a good worker, but he was dead inside . Eventually we drifted apart but he will still every once in a while call me to see how its going. I always ask if he's been able to lick the booze and his depression but he always says everything is the same. He has a great sadness in his voice. If his girls would only realize the job they did on him. He needs to go away for some extended drying out and therapy and then he would make some lucky girl a great guy!

There were five or six guys that I dated that I only had a couple of dates apiece with. At the time, that I met them, I thought they were what I was looking for, but after a couple of dates I knew better. If you give it a couple of dates, and nothing is happening in the chemistry department its better to call it off right then and there. The longer you try and let it go on the harder it becomes, especially if he starts making noises like your the one for him!

I have a history of staying with a guy out of pity, it's not a smart thing. I have a real hard time breaking up with a guy who really wants a relationship with me and is doing all the right things to please me. I have had that happen to me, and I don't want to be the one to inflict the hurt. Sometimes its necessary, and its better to do it at the beginning then to go out together for months, and then do it. The longer you go on, the harder it is to break it off.

So, as soon as you know its not working, be merciful and break it off. For instance, One guy I met, who worked on the big dig in Boston, his name was also John. I was at the Village one night, he was standing at the end of the bar. I thought he was extremely good looking, he was talking to another girl. As a contest, I told my girl friend, see that guy? She said yes, I said I can make him come ask me to dance without speaking to him, or without getting off my stool. She laughed, I started just staring at him, even though he was not looking at me. In a few minutes he looked up. When he did I smiled sweetly and then dropped my eyes to my drink and sipped my straw. Then I looked his way again, he looked up, I smiled again but this time held his eyes with mine. I continued this play for a very short time. Then he excused himself from the other girl and came over and asked me to dance.

We danced together for the rest of the night, he asked me out and took my phone number. He came down that weekend and we went out. We walked all over Portsmouth, and hit every restaurant and bar in the town. We laughed our asses off. He told me he owned property in Boston and Florida, we seemed to be fairly compatible. He said he was going to work another five years and retire. He said I was the type of woman he wanted to retire with. He was extremely handsome, and was very tanned from working outside all the time. He had a fantastic body, from doing all the heavy work he did. He had white curly hair, and a small moustache, which looked great in contrast to his tanned skin. He came down during the week, only this time he didn't want to go out. He sent me to the supermarket for snacks and beer. He ate and drank and fell asleep on my sofa. Woke up in a couple hours and went home.

We went out maybe two more times, but I realized, he drank too much, and was a bit selfish. Then after not seeing him for a week or two, I saw him at a dance with another woman. I didn't care that he was there with another woman, but he tried to ignore me. He cautiously waved at me behind her back, I did not like that. The next time he called, I told him. All he had to do was say Hi and introduce me. He said she wouldn't like that, she would be jealous. I broke it off. I refused to go out with him again. He called three or four more times but each time I told him no, I was busy. Three years later he still tries to get me to go out with him but I always refuse.

I always encourage my girlfriends, if your interested in a particular guy you need to go ask them to dance, or use that little trick if your afraid to go ask them. Guys are very afraid of rejection, and if you ask them, they will usually stay with you for the rest of the night. Sometimes you can't get rid of them.

The saga of my John's , continues there were two more Johns, one was a tall very young looking, handsome, sensitive face. He worked at the Race Track. He was very taken with me. He insisted he was forty-nine years old, but he looked twenty-eight. He has been after me for three years I dance with him, we have become friends as far as conversation goes, but the chemistry is not there. And finally a fourth John, he was a hot shit, I met one night at the Ashworth. Long hair in back, but receding in front. Great dancer and great personality. He danced with me all night several times both there, and another place downtown. We went to breakfast a couple of times. He asked me out several times. Good job, but I know he has another girl friend, and I don't want to get involved so he is also someone I dance with and talk to and have a good time with but no relationship or ever chance of one.

Not too long after I had first began going to the Village on Friday and Saturday nights right after I had broken up with Mike, I was sitting there on my favorite stool, and this little ball of energy comes charging in. He came up to the end of the bar like gangbusters. Small, nervous little bundle of energy. Salt and pepper curly hair, full moustache, and kind of poppy eyes, like Gregory Hines. His eyes were a lot like my old friend Sam's. At first I wasn't impressed, he was smoking and I hate that. He had a wonderful smile, and dimples, and I love that. He came on strong and offered to buy me a drink. I accepted, we started talking, he asked me to dance. He was a great dancer and you could tell he loved it. Not too many guys love to dance. They will dance to please a lady, but if they love it its a bonus, because you know they will continue to do it, even after you start going out with them. He sang when he danced which I do too, and we had a ball. We danced together all night, and by the end of the evening knew a lot about each other. He kept hugging and kissing me, on the face, neck side of the head, hand anywhere. We were all over the floor, singing dancing and laughing. I found out he was only forty-eight, never married and coming off a five-year relationship.

He said he was in no hurry to get back into another relationship and I told him he was perfect for me because neither did I. He took my phone number, I told him I was living out of my car on weekends and that I was staying at my youngest daughters that night. When I got back to my daughters, I had just walked into the house, when the phone rang. It was Al and I sat down on the kitchen floor with the phone and we talked for another two hours. We seemed to be totally smitten with one another.

The following week he called me every night, and we talked well over an hour each night. We were like a couple of school kids. Finally he made a date for the following weekend. He and his buddy, Warren came down to Portsmouth. We went out to eat and then dancing. We wound up going to a place the young people go to dance. It was called Banana's, my oldest daughter and her girl friends were there that night. I introduced them all to Al, he was a big hit. He spent money like it was water, buying drinks for all the kids.

We raised hell, he kept telling the kids how wonderful I was. We were really beginning to fall for one another and we mugged up all night. His friend had a great time dancing with all the young girls and when the place closed we all went to Breakfast. Then we closed up a couple of other nightclubs and they started for home, about 3:00 am. The following week I didn't hear from him at all. I couldn't understand what had gone wrong. I went to the Village on the weekend and he wasn't there. Then I heard he had gone to Florida for a week, he hadn't told me he was going to Florida. When I finally saw him again, a couple of weeks had gone by. I spotted Warren first.

I had a policy of not giving a guy a hard time, if they didn't call me, but considering the first week I was really stymied as to what had happened to change things. The last thing they had said to me, was what a fantastic time they had. The excuse was, Al was falling for me, and he did not want to get into a new relationship so fast after the old one, so his solution was stay away. In Warren's words he was falling hard and fast so he ran. I looked right at Warren and said, well you know what "Fuck Al", if he can't talk to me and tell me he wants to cool it or whatever.

Half way through the evening Al came over. He said Warren had told him what I had said. I said Yes, if that's the way you felt you could have had the decency to come over and tell me you want to cool it for a while or something, not just ignore me like I did something.

We danced again, and he was just as affectionate, but I had cooled a little. After that our relationship sort of turned into a little love, hate relationship. We dated about once a month, when we did date, we had a hell of a time and it lasted two days. Then we wouldn't date again for another month.

Mean while we would see each other at the Village and dance with each other a few times, but I was also dating others and dancing with them. We seemed to have an understanding about our relationship, neither of us really wanted to look at a long-term relationship so soon. The difference between he and I however, his method of not getting involved, was to close himself off to all feelings, and possibilities. Even though I was not looking for a husband or a long-term relationship, I was always open to whatever might happen. You have to be, unless you want to take the chance of losing the one good thing that might happen to you if you were open to it.

Things happen when we least expect it, and many people have ruined their lives by being closed, and keeping their emotions and feelings to themselves, because they don't want to get hurt again. No one wants to get hurt. But unless you are open, you will miss out on a lot of great things. Al, was so intent on not getting involved again that he would not let his feelings take control. You could see the turmoil in him. Many times during our relationship, he would be ready to let himself go, but would back off. Once or twice when he was feeling good and without thinking he told me he loved me. Then he caught himself and changed the subject, instead he would say, he admired me, or he was crazy about me. You could tell he didn't like my going out with other men, but he didn't want to give me any more time. Our dates would be grand plans, when he would really try to impress me, they would start with a $40.00 bottle of wine, followed by a grand dinner in an exclusive place. Maybe dinner music. Then off for dancing at some ballroom, and then off to some intimate little place for desert and nightcaps. Maybe breakfast. In six months we had maybe four or five of those dates, all grand all fun. I liked him a lot, and if he had been more demanding of my time, could have fallen for him. We would talk on the phone a lot, but not as much as the first week. He loved my kids and always asked for them, he saw them as much as he could when he was around, and maybe attended four or five parties where they were.

My kids threw me a wonderful surprise 60th birthday party, they didn't know whom I was going out with the most so they invited five of my boyfriends, four showed up and the only reason the others didn't was because they were working. The guys all got along great even though they were all trying to be my one and only.

One night I was at my regular Tuesday night hang out, Pazzaluna. I was sitting at the middle bar where I always sat with my girlfriends. I always went to Pazzaluna with the girls or by myself, never with a date. It was a singles, and they always gave you a free hot buffet, had great music, and it was smaller and more intimate than the Village.

All of a sudden, this adorable, handsome small Italian man came up behind my stool and started talking to me. His name was Tony, he had dark curly hair and he was adorable. He asked me to dance. He loved dancing, and we wound up dancing together all night. We talked a lot, we had a lot in common. He was the only man I had met who was almost my age. He was one year younger. He had boundless energy, he had a beauty shop he owned and he worked as a bartender part time. He had been married twice for nearly as long as I had. He had five children, as I did and we just seemed to hit it off beautifully. The problem was, at the time I was already seeing about three guys and I really didn't think I could handle another one, so for sometime our relationship consisted of dancing together at Pazzaluna. Then one night we were talking, and I mentioned a club I enjoyed in Portsmouth on a Thursday night. He said it sounded like great fun and he would love to come down and go with me. I gave in, and the following week he came down. We went to the club and had dinner and listened to jazz and danced. He was very romantic, and hard to resist, I liked him a lot.

He was sweet and caring, he absolutely loved to dance, as much as I did. That was unusual for a man, most men danced to please a woman but they did not really enjoy it. Tony did, we danced well together. The chemistry was fantastic. He began coming to Portsmouth at least twice a week, we were becoming a couple and were very smitten with each other. We would go out to the jazz clubs during the week and on Sunday would walk around down town. He never stayed over night, he had two daughters still living at home and he was very aware of getting home every night. I worried about his driving back late, and a couple of times he did have a close call. We had both told each other at the beginning of our relationship that we did not want to get remarried or get into a long term relationship we both understood that the other one could date other people, if they wished. I don't think that Tony was, however. I say that only because, a couple of times when he just went to a party without me, he would, "confess" that he had been out without me. I was continuing to see a couple of other men at the same time. He was very generous, but I could see that the longer it went on, the harder it was for him to come so far to see me. He would work till 6:30 go home change drive the 60 miles or so to my house, go downtown to a nice restaurant, have a great evening and then drive all the way home.

One night he got a ticket for speeding, another he got stopped, because his car was swerving from one lane to another. I was afraid he was going to fall asleep at the wheel and I think he was afraid of that too. He never complained, but I could tell it was wearing on him. He would have preferred to spend more time on the weekends with me, but I was dating Jim at the time and the weekends were his.

Once when I went to his hometown to meet him, we had a great supper at a super Italian restaurant. After supper we went back to his place. His youngest daughter, whom he was supposed to be picking up at work at 11:00 came strolling in earlier, and practically caught us in the middle of something. His daughter was irate that he had a woman there, and instead of telling her off, in a nice way. He allowed her to tell him off. I knew then, that as much as he cared for me, his daughters would always be more important. Even though I had no aspirations of getting married or anything, I have to be number one to the man I am having a relationship with, if I am going to be monogamous. Tony and I were great friends as well as lovers, and it would be hard to break it off. We had been going out more than six months, and totally the opposite from Al, when you were with Tony he gave you his undivided attention. He made me feel like a Queen, and to this day we are still the best of friends, and I hope always will be. I dated no losers, if I went out with them once and found they had problems, that was it. Don't expect them to change, no one does.

Naturally like anyone, I did meet a lot of jerks, or guys who are out for one thing. They are generally easy to detect, if you're on your toes.

Most of the guys out there, are really nice, decent guys, and I considered myself extremely lucky that so many of them were attracted to me. I would meet lots of girls, who would sit and complain, that they had been going to the singles for two years and had never met one nice guy. Well, if that's true you better look in the mirror, your either a bitch, a whiner, or both. You need to think about what you're doing wrong if that's the case.

Another time, I was on the dance floor at the Village. I looked up to see a tall attractive, curly haired man starring at me. I smiled, and when I came off the floor, he and a friend came over to me. He smiled and said, my friend and I have been watching you for several weeks. We wanted to approach you, but you always seem to have several men around you.

This is the first time we have been able to catch you alone, and they introduced themselves, and told me they were both in love with me.

I was very flattered, the tall attractive one asked me to dance, his name was Dennis. We danced for the remainder of the night and he asked me out. Although he was in his early fifties, he was retired. He made his living on investment properties. He had one son, and plenty of time. He began coming down to Portsmouth on Monday nights and taking me out to dinner. He was very interested in History and loved to roam the really old buildings, restaurants and houses in Portsmouth. He was extremely interesting to talk to and our dinners were always very informative. Over the summer we went to all the great restaurants in the area, he would always read all the information about the building displayed on the walls, or on the menus. He was sweet and quiet and good company. He always dressed well, and money was no object. He was an ardent lover and we got along very well for about three months, before I broke up with him to go steady with Jim.

Jim is our next story. Toward the end of the summer, after spending most of that summer with Tony, Dennis, John, Al, Mike and numerous other single dates, I was at the Village one night. It was almost the end of the evening, I had been there with Rachel and we had a very good time as usual. A small dark haired man, leaned across me to get a drink at the bar. He was trying in vain to get the bartenders attention. I looked up at him, and asked if he would like some help. He smiled at me, and when he smiled, his whole face lit up with the most gorgeous dimples, I had ever seen. I commented, Oh you have beautiful dimples! He smiled even broader, Oh thank you what else do you like about me? I said, not a dam thing, just your dimples. He laughed, he apparently liked my sense of humor. He stayed and we started talking, the evening was almost over, but we talked for a while. He was very funny and easy to talk to, but I was not particularly attracted to him.

Besides, I had enough boyfriends and didn't want anymore! He was totally charming however, and included Rachel in the conversation. When we went to the car he followed us and asked for my number.

The following Monday I was at work, and my phone rang. It was him Jim, he said what time do you get home from work? I told him, he said I will be standing on your doorstep, with a bouquet of Roses to take you to dinner.

I got home and there he was. How could you argue with that? We had a great dinner, and he stayed and we made love that very night. It was great. I began seeing him on a regular basis, because he had kids still at home and worked a really odd shift in Boston, he had to come on Friday and Saturday. I still saw the other guys during the week, but weekends became Jims. The more I saw of him the better friends we became.

At the beginning of our relationship I had no intention of getting any more involved with him than I did any of the others, in fact on a one to ten basis he would have not even been in the top three. The more I saw of him, however the more he worked his way into my life. He was different from the others, in that he did not take me on expensive dates, he did not make love and disappear, he did not avoid meeting my family, or talking about the future. He would take me on dates like, a trip up the mountains for the day to enjoy the foliage. An early morning walk on the beach. A day in Boston just walking around and enjoying one of the feasts at the North End. He took me to his house for the weekend and introduced me to his kids, his mother, and his family. He invited me to family weddings, and introduced me to his personal friends. He listened to my advice about his kids or his house. He asked my opinion in how to buy new clothes. Slowly but surely he began to get an edge. We had a lot in common, our sense of humor, our general good nature, our kids, what we liked to do. He didn't mind going shopping he enjoyed my friends. We were constantly laughing. We went sailing and hot air ballooning. He took me on a golf weekend with his friends. We both loved movies. His imagination was wonderful, while the other guys were sending me roses, he would bake me an apple pie from scratch. If he ever heard me say I liked something the next weekend he would show up with it. For instance one Sunday we were cooking breakfast, I said I would like a bacon press to put on the English muffins. The next week a bacon press arrived in the mail ! Another time, I mentioned that when I lived in

Wolfeboro, I loved the lemon Bismarck's they made at that Duncan Donuts. The next week he went to an Italian bakery in Billerica and had them make me some lemon Bismarck's. Another time he installed a bulletin board in my exercise room. On the top it said "Why I love Effie", he would hang little post-its on the board every once in a while with the reasons. Eventually it was full. After a couple of months, he broke it off with any other girls he was going with. I was flattered but I told him I was not ready to do that yet.

I thought and thought about it, but I had only been single a little over a year, I was not ready to go steady again, I was having too good a time.

Over the next couple of months, Jim started spending more and more time at my house. Besides the weekend, he would be down one or two extra nights during the week. I'm sure he was trying to work the other guys out of my life, and he figured the more nights he was there the less I would be able to see them. It did make it harder but I was not ready to commit to one person. It was a real burden to him, besides having the grown kids at home he had to police. He had to be at work by 5:00 am, so I would get up with him around 3 get his breakfast, pack his lunch, give him coffee, send him out the door and go back to bed.

As it got to be winter, it was even harder. Then after we had been going out maybe six months or so, several things happened that began to change my mind. That Christmas, he was the one that really spent a lot of time with me. We helped each other decorate our trees, we spent time with both his family and mine.

Tony came down for an evening and brought me a nice gift, but he spent his holiday with his kids and ex wife and did not invite me. Mike, stayed sober long enough to come to my family with me on Christmas Eve, and I went to his house long enough to open gifts with him. The others I did not see. Jim spent the better part of the Holidays with me. Jim was very tolerant of Mike who often was a real pain in the ass. When he was drinking, he would often call my house ten or twelve times in a single night, and say the same things over and over. I never lied to Jim, I always told him who it was and what he wanted. He began to kid about it and call him our oldest son! We felt sorry for him, but at the same time he was really making our lives hell. Sometimes he would cry and say what did I ever do to you, to have you treat me so mean.? and I would try to explain to him, that I was not being mean, that I needed him to get well and get sober and make a life for himself, but it fell on deaf ears. New Years, I planned to go out with Al, I really wanted to do something special and Jim had only mentioned going to the Village. He was disappointed, but I really wanted a good time. It turned out to be not quite so good. He took me into Boston, we got a room in a hotel. We had dinner in a great restaurant that was all decorated up for New Years. I was a big hit with his friends etc. but as Al always did, he floated from place to place leaving me alone half the time. When I took up with two fellows at the bar who were doing magic tricks, he saw red. We had a big fight about it. In the end, he said I was right and he apologized. We did have a good time dancing after that, but I guess I could see he was always going to be the playboy. We stayed over at the Hotel but we didn't have sex or anything, and in the morning we went right home.

Jim was upset that I had spent New Years with Al, he knew him, and he wasn't his favorite person. Of course he had no idea, even though I told him what had gone on.

A week or so after New Years, I had an operation on my foot. I had told all the guys that this was going to happen. Tony said, don't worry we'll go to the piano bar and sing if you can't dance. Mike was concerned, but Jim was the one who was there for me. I had let everyone at the Village know I would not be there for a month or so.

The day of the operation, there was a bad snowstorm. It was o.k. early in the morning when I first went. My daughter in law came to pick me up, and got my medicines and made me comfortable at my condo, a girl friend came down and kept me company for most of the afternoon. As the weather began to get worse, she went home. Jim called from Boston and said he was coming as soon as work got out. He called me from his house after work, by that time it had taken him two hours to get to his home from Boston. I told him don't even try to come down, it was too dangerous. I told him I was perfectly comfortable and he could wait till the next day or till the snow was cleared. He also had to be sure his daughter got home from Boston safely. He was going to pick her up at the train. He thanked me for understanding. I fell asleep on my couch, about 11:30 p.m. I heard the door, he had come down! It wasn't fit for man or beast but he had come. He stayed all weekend. The next day in the deep snow, he lugged me out to get my nails done, and waited for me at the Beauty parlor. The following day he took me to get my hair done and waited again. I had my bad foot wrapped in a plastic bag! He took me out to dinner and waited on me hand and foot. Tony and Mike both called to see how I was, but it ended there. Jim spent every minute he could with me over the next four to six weeks, helping whenever I needed him.

So shortly after that when he told me he could no longer stand to share me with anyone else. That he loved me and wanted me to be his, exclusively, I had to give it serious consideration. I told him finally that I would try. I was not convinced myself that it was the best thing for me, I did not want to give up Tony and Dennis, and Al. I thought about it a long time. I wasn't sure I could give up my fantastic single life. I loved him, but I wasn't sure how much. I thought I loved Tony and Al. I had never in my life been so popular, not even when I was a teenager, or when I was divorced at forty. It was a dream come true for me. I was sixty years old, I would never have another chance. I was also concerned about his life. He still had kids at home, was he going to be able to give me the attention I wanted? Three of his kids were still living at home, one was getting ready to move out but the other two were eighteen and twenty. His home was over fifty miles from mine. I would have preferred to leave things as they were for a couple of more years. I knew he couldn't do that, it tore him up.

I thought about the others, I knew Al would never settle down, but I didn't want to settle down, he could take me the places I wanted to go, he loved to raise hell the same as I did. He had never been married so there were no ex wives or kids to compete with. I knew Tony didn't want to settle down, and he was so totally into his daughters, I would always be second fiddle.

I thought about how close Jim and I had become, the truly wonderful things he said to me every single day. He told me he never felt the way he did about me about anyone ever. Not his wife, no one. Then he told me, how he first knew for sure he was in love with me, and I thought how many guys would say something like that. Most guys, won't even tell you, they love you, let alone go into a whole story about it. This is what he told me, and he wrote it down, so I can never forget it.

One night we were at the Village, it was just after a holiday, and we hadn't been out for a couple of weeks. We were all dying to get out. It was one of the coldest nights of the year. We went with Rachel. We were only there a little while, when the electricity went out. We all sat in candlelight for an hour or so waiting for it to come back on, but it never did. Then everybody started talking about where we should go next. Some were going to Natalies, some to Pazzaluna, we decided to go to the Ashworth. Jim said he would get the car, Rachel and I started outside. Rachel slipped and fell on the walk and hurt her back. I helped her inside and to a chair. Jim got the car but when he got to it, it had a flat tire. I went outside with him, to help him change it. He was in a suit and tie, I was in an evening gown. It had to be at least 5o below zero. I tried to get him to call AAA but he said it would take too long he would change it. I stayed with him helping him get the tools etc. We had a hell of a time getting the tire out, I have a big Caddy and the tire is secured in the back of the trunk. You have to practically climb into the trunk to get it. We both squatted down on the ground to put the tire on. Jim was doing all the physical labor but I was doing what I could to help. Jim's hand were freezing, but he never complained, he said he looked over and there I was squatting next to him smiling at him, and at that moment he knew for sure he loved me. ! He said any other girl would have been in the warm building waiting for him to finish, but I stayed with him freezing in the cold!! Giving him company and support. When he told me that, I knew I had to give him a chance, not other man had ever spoken to me, from the heart as he did.

HOW TO BE HOT AT SIXTY

The following week, I told first Al, and then Tony and Dennis and Mike and John, that I was going steady and could no longer date. They were flabbergasted. Tony was sad, he didn't say much, just you do what you have to do. He stayed close friends with both of us. Jim liked him. Al said your crazy, you don't want to settle down, you're just like me ! The others just congratulated me and were true gentlemen. If I see them we speak, we're friendly.

Jim and I did have an understanding that, we would still go to the singles with our friends. That we would not be jealous if either of us danced with a friend. That we would continue to be social . I told him I could not put up with jealousy, if he started acting possessive it would be the end.

At first I thought, it was the end of an era, my life would never be the same again. Through the spring and summer we went "steady". It was kind of trial and error for us. We had a lot to learn about each other, and a lot was happening in our lives. Jim's life was changing rapidly, almost too rapidly, he had sort of planned on keeping his house for another year or two. When his youngest daughter moved out unexpectedly that summer, and his youngest son went to school in the fall, (off to college). He had some major empty nest feelings. His wife had walked out on him six years before, leaving him with four children. His life had been pretty much the kids for those six years, and now they were all gone. To make matters worse he had a balloon mortgage payment come do and the ex would not sign to extend it, so he was forced to sell the house. It was a huge evolvement for him. I think it affected him more than he could really tell at the time. I was not the one causing any of this, but trying to establish a new relationship and deal with all of these issues was very difficult. He had gotten himself into deep debt in college loans for the kids. His ex was a jealous, bitter woman, and she would not help him at all with any of the kids school bills. When he told the youngest daughter she would have to go to an less expensive school that year, she got angry with him and moved in with her mother, which broke his heart. He was over $90,000.00 in debt between school loans and a second mortgage he had no choice. I helped him fix the house up to sell. We spent many weekends there cleaning stuff out, I think even though none of this was my fault, I think the kids connected his starting a relationship with me with his selling the house.

I got along ok with two of them but the other two were very cold to me. All this was extra pressure and stress on Jim. At first he seemed to be handling it ok but every once in a while, I think he would think about it and maybe feel he was rushing the kids out of the house or something, because his mood would change and you could tell something was bothering him.

If we talked about it, and he let me know what was wrong we could work through it, but he wasn't used to talking about his feelings and it was hard sometimes to read him. The situation would have been the same for him, whether I was in the picture or not. It was a natural progression, of children going off to school, or growing up and moving out on their own.

However, because I had come into the picture at the same time, he needed to be sure in his own mind, that he was not causing them to move prematurely. The hidden tension, made it easier to blow things out of proportion. One week end in the summer, after we had been going steady for about six months, I was having a surprise 40th birthday for my oldest daughter.

He said he couldn't come because he had a golf weekend, the second one that summer. In the meantime, Mike was on another dry out, where he hadn't had any booze for a month or so and was doing really well. He was still calling me and had asked me to go to Boston for the weekend. I had said no, but when Jim went away with the guys to play golf instead of coming to my daughters party I was very tempted. Then he found out the golf weekend was the following weekend, but he was going to go check out a college with his son that weekend and play golf the following.

We were fighting, he was tense, he was beginning to talk like he wanted to put off selling the house for another year, etc. I told him I did not have the time to wait a couple of years for him to be ready for a relationship. I was sixty-one years old, I needed to enjoy myself now. I wound up going to Boston with Mike while he went to play golf. It was a mistake, but I think in the end it helped our relationship. I had a wonderful weekend, Mike was better than I had ever seen him. He was clean, sober, his intellect was sharp. We walked all through Harvard, and he told me everything about the place. He knew Boston like the back of his hand and he knew about every building. It was fun and informative. He took me out to dinner, at two wonderful exclusive restaurants. We went dancing. We went to the gay pride parade. We went shopping. He was a perfect gentleman, and while I was impressed and still had some feelings for him, I made no promises.

When I got back, there was a nasty note from Jim and all his stuff had been cleared out of my house. He even called Mike and talked bad about me, and told him he could have me. I didn't want Mike, I was trying to help him stay sober, but I thought maybe it was for the best. I tried, it didn't work. I didn't hear from Jim for maybe two weeks. I didn't really resume my dating. I went to the Village and danced but I spent my weekends up in Wolfeboro with friends.

I did see Mike one more time, but he had not really given up the booze. He was sick most of the time. He had been wonderful in Boston, but the minute he was home he went right back to it.

After about two weeks, I spoke to Jim on the phone, because we had made some plans together that needed to be addressed. We were going away on a golf weekend with his friends, we had the hot air balloon tickets, and we had planned to go to Las Vegas in the winter. We had both put money into a lot of this stuff and had two tickets to everything. He called to see if I knew anyone who would buy his tickets. I told him I didn't. Then I tried to explain to him my side of the situation, but he was not interested. I told him there was no reason we could not go on the balloon ride together even though we were not going out any more. He did agree to that. I think the minute we started talking to each other on the phone, we both knew we would have to get back together, but we had said somethings that needed resolving. I told him I was going to the Palace dancing that night, he said he might be there.

He showed up that night, and when I saw him I was amazed. He had lost at least twenty pounds in the two weeks. I later found out he had been in terrible shape, not eating, crying, sick. I hated myself for doing that to him, when I saw him I hugged him, and that was it. We talked it out, it was hard getting him to do that, I was a talker, he was a brooder. We were back together, and we have never been out of each others sight since.

As the relationship resumed we were closer than ever, he had a key to my place and he began spending all his time there. Especially after September when his last child moved out. He found he couldn't stand to be in the empty house. It made it easier to put it on the market.

We continued to work there every weekend to clean the place out and get it ready. His ex was a major problem, because she wanted her share of the money for the house, but she wasn't ready to sign anything or help in any way. We became closer and closer however, he would leave me sweet little notes everywhere, in my lunch, in the mailbox, on my car seat.

At the end of September he retired from driving the bus, and he moved down that very day. I came home from work, on my front door was a big note. The note said, I have three presents for you, if you can guess the first two, you can have the last one. I opened the door, (my condo is on the second floor, so there are stairs as you come in). On the stairs was another note and a lot of floating balloons, one big helium fancy balloon said, this is the first present.

The smell of roasting turkey filled my nostrils, turkey is my favorite meal! As I ascended the stairs, I could see the table beautifully decorated and a huge turkey roasted in the middle! I yelled oh my gosh, turkey! He yelled, you guessed the second present! He grabbed me and hugged me, and led me to my seat, he said now you get the third present. He put a beautiful blue velvet little trunk in front of me. I opened the lid, and inside was a gorgeous red velvet box, and inside of that, a set of rings. It was a beautiful set I had seen in Boston, I had showed it to him, just non-chalantly one-day when we were window-shopping. At the time I had said, I never intend to get married, but if I ever did that would be the ring I would want.

He had bought it! I was really flabbergasted, I did not want a ring and had not intended to become engaged but it was a wonderful surprise. He told me all the reasons he had decided to get it, and how apprehensive he had been as well. It was from the heart and so sweet, I accepted it. I wear it constantly, but I am still not sure I will get married.

It has now as I am writing this, been another year, and we get along better and better all the time. People have accepted us as a couple and some even call him my husband, but so far I have not seen any reason to our benefits to take that final step. We still go to the singles and associate with our friends we met there, including my old boy friends.

Tony is still a good friend to us both. This weekend for instance we are going to Tony's sixtieth birthday party. Al has become a sort of recluse, I think he is regretting not making commitments to someone. Warren his friend has matured more and become more of a friend to us. John the widow is still not well, and drinking too much, John from the big dig has turned into a drunk, we see him every week at the dances and he is always alone, and staggering. Mike, after a year of hard drinking, and sickness, and accidents, and not taking his medications, etc. was found dead Holy Saturday morning by a neighbor. We were very very sad about this but we did all we could for him. It saddens us that so nice a guy, could be brought so low by abuse of a substance that he could have controlled if he just got the help. Its such a waste. We know he is at peace, and that the demons can no longer get to him.

We have met many more single people our age that we have a great time with and who are fun people and loyal friends. We dance with others if we feel we want to, if Jim is working he doesn't mind my going out with my girl friends. He still plays golf at least once a week with the guys. I have taken it up and we play with other couples other times. He still takes his annual weeklong golf trip with the guys. We have taken three trips together and had great time. The house finally sold, we paid off all his college debt. The minute it did, his ex wife took him to court for child support, even though the two kids still in college don't even live with her, their official mailing address is her house. We pay her $800.00 a month support. She got $80,000.00 from the house.

Jim walked away with nothing after paying the college debts off. We don't care, we see the light at the end of the tunnel, and when the kids are out of college in three years he will be free and know he did the right thing. She will be alone, bitter, and unhappy, because you can't ever be happy when you are so vindictive. We enjoy talking to people our age, and showing them their is life after divorce and old age!

We have taken a lot of people out with us and introduced them around, we are responsible for a few good connections. You are never too old, this year alone we fixed up an eighty one year old lady who was miserable and depressed with an eighty one year old widowed millionaire from Puerto Rico. He took her to Florida, and Puerto Rico, and gave her money and showed her a grand time. In the end after a few months it did not work out, because he wanted sex too often for her.! She had her chance though, we thought he was great fun and a hot ticket.

I had spent the day with him, when he came in from Puerto Rico. He took me for lunch, that night Jim and I took him to the Ashworth, dancing. He kept telling us he hadn't danced since prep school, but by the end of the evening he was making the rounds, asking all the attractive older ladies to dance. He had a ball. He is not living in Florida and has found a lady friend.

We introduced another sixty seven year old lady friend of ours, to an attractive fifty four year old man we knew. They hit it off terrifically and are going steady and having a grand time. We also talked two of Jims retired friends from work, into going to the singles, and now they are their three times a week along with us. Its their social life and it really keeps them in the swing of things. They are both in their middle to late fifties, very shy and self conscious, but we introduced them around. I danced with them for a while, until we could give them some confidence, now they circulate like they'd been doing it forever. We have done this a lot, with friends or even strangers that we meet who are lonely, or depressed and don't know how to make a change in their lives. We generally have great success in turning them around and giving them a new lease on life. They get renewed interest in socializing, in dressing up and getting out and getting exercise. We now have our own crowd of about twenty that hand around together and just have a ball.

Things do not change, we change: (Henry Thoreau 1817-1862 American essayist & poet.

Chapter nine:

"What's Hot?"

Hot is a new expression that the kids use to express sexy. When we say, How to be "Hot at sixty," we are not just talking about hot sexually. We are using "Hot" to describe a feeling of well being. There are a lot more factors, than sexual, that go into making you "Hot". It is more than just physical or sexual feelings. Being "Hot" is a whole attitude, its a whole way of life. Every facet of your life has to be alive, vital, healthy.

My fiancée and I were just discussing the other night, what exactly is the basic difference between the people our age that are exciting, healthy and youthful human beings, and the ones who are over weight, unhealthy, dull and depressed. (In defense of some, over weight people, I am not intimating that every one who is over weight, is unhealthy, but it is a fact that along with advanced age, and becoming sedentary, most people do get way out of shape, and very over weight.) Nuf said.

The main reason is you have to continue as you grow older to want to find new and exciting things to do every day. You have to continue to grow, to have goals, to have a reason to get out of bed and to continue in that tedious job. You have to want to change and grow, no matter how old you become.

When I was younger, I had a goal, that every single year, I would learn something new. One year it was belly dancing, another yoga, but always something. I just saw on television yesterday, a man who is still a busboy at a major hotel, at ninety years old. I could not believe how great and youthful he was. He could still throw a heavy suitcase onto a pile of luggage. He spoke with a firm strong voice, he walked with a firm steady gait. He loved going to work and socializing every day.

It's wonderful to be able to retire, it's great to "grow old gracefully". That does not mean, job well done, I'm content to spend my remaining years sitting on the porch watching the grandchildren. My life is basically over. If that's your attitude, then it is! Over weight, bad eating habits, drinking too much, smoking, and being sedentary, are very bad for you, and they work off one another. The longer you sit, and eat, and rest, the more content you become. Until your always tired, no energy, couch potato's. If the most exciting thing you do for a night out is go out to dinner, your doomed. If going to parties and socializing is not your thing, and you really enjoy baby sitting the grandchildren every Friday and Saturday night, make it fun and exciting. Take the kids, skating, biking, hiking, bowling but don't sit in the house watching television while they play computer games. Make Grandma, exciting and fun. My grandkids love miniature golf, swimming, tubing, dancing. When my oldest grand daughter was two, I used to bring my tap shoes over her house and we would tap dance on her toy box.

Many grandparents, think this is the way they are supposed to live, because their grandparents did it that way. Oh no, we haven't danced in ten years, I need my beauty sleep, if I don't get eight hours, I'm no good the next day!

Grandparents today are youthful, they work much later in life. Some start a brand new career after they retire. Energy begets energy, get a job, go dancing, walking, hiking you will find renewed energy. You'll be saying I never felt so good in my life.

If your alone, divorced, widowed, single, try the singles clubs. When we looked around the singles on Saturday night, of the 500 or so people there, mostly over forty, their are probably less than 10% of them that are over weight. Compare that to the people you see going out to dinner, or walking around the malls, or most any other place you see lots of people today. Its not because they go to the singles, its because they are out exercising, and socializing. They are getting on with life. They are active people.

Exercising is something you do extra, if you get exercise on your job, great but as you get older you need to do extra things to exercise. Dancing, hiking, jogging, golf (without the cart), bowling, biking, swimming, rollerblading, skating, aerobics, all of the above. Everyone can do at least two of those things. An occasional thing doesn't cut it, do something at least two or three times a week, scheduled activities and regulating your diet, will make you "Hot". If you don't take control of your life, and make it your life, and what you really want to do at fifty or sixty, when you get to seventy you'll be going through a whole new crisis. Your children will be looking for the "Home". The grandchildren will be outgrowing you, and you'll be sitting there alone again only older and fatter, and more unhealthy than you were at fifty.

Whether you want a lifetime companion, or just a dinner and dancing Saturday night partner, its healthy to establish a relationship from many standpoints. You need adult conversation, the grandchildren may be fun, but you need to talk about current events, or other adult subjects. You need the flirtation, compliments, and validation from a member of the opposite sex once in a while, or even from your own sex. I kid with my girlfriends, that men are only good for three things, sex, dancing and fixing things. Even if that were really your attitude, you need them for those things. Even if you only need them for one thing, that's one thing you need. Readers digest had a great article last year on how sex keeps you youthful. They had scientific proof, that your hormones have to be on the move, that orgasms are the fountain of youth. Look around you at the people you know get it and make your own comparisons. We just heard on television tonight, that they are recommending the Boston marathon runners have sex the night before. If they want to run their best race!

I just read an article by Dr. David Weeks, a neuropsychologist at the Royal Edinburgh Hospital. It says sex at least three times a week, can make people look and feel at least ten years younger. Another study done on the strength of the immune system, which found that those who had sex at least two times a week, had one third higher levels of LGA a substance that helps the body fight off colds and viruses.

To be "Hot", every fiber of your body has to be at peak performance. You need a reason to get up every day. You need to look forward to everyday. When you jump out of bed in the morning, (and you should jump not roll), You need to be able to say, oh great today I'm doing this, or that.

I have a very good friend, a gentleman, who retired, about five years ago, from a very physical job. Up to that point, in his late fifties, he was very fit, attractive, and tan. He had been divorced some years before, and had been looking for a lady. He used mainly the personal adds, which is o.k. and very successful for a lot of people. For him face to face would have been better, because he was so fussy! He wanted someone who looked like a model, but who would love to go fishing, and hunting and staying in a cabin in the woods. He wanted a gorgeous face, great body, no extra weight, sophisticated, yet she should love to clean fish, and roam in the woods. He lives in the mountains and she would have to love that. He hates coming to the city. Needless to say he did not find one. We introduced him to several nice ladies, but one was too fat, and one too expensive etc.

Now he's sort of given up, he just had a knee operation, he sits around home entertaining his grandchildren and telling me how happy he is. However when the grandchildren are home, or doing their own thing, he gets drunk and calls me and cries on my shoulder. When his son's have the time between their jobs, and families, they come up and go hunting with him etc. but more time than not they have their own lives and don't have the time. So two or three times a week I can expect a call from him, drunk, telling me stories of his grandkids and how crazy he is about them. How much greater it would have been if he had settled for a nice companion that would keep him company, even if she is ten pounds over weight. He is only going to get worse as he gets older, and will probably be a real pain in the ass to his kids in a few years. I try to talk him into coming to Portsmouth and going out to the singles with us, but he says its too far, its maybe fifty miles. He wants me to come there, but without my fiancée! He is a great guy, he has a lot to offer, but he needs to change a little. Compromise, if the only thing wrong with the gal is a couple of pounds he can help her take it off.

Give a real girl a chance, or a guy. Think about your life, what is good and what is bad with it? Keep the good, throw the bad away and start over. Substitute the bad with something that's more fulfilling. Don't think of anything as unattainable. Also look at things realistically though. You can attain almost anything, but if your a cripple your not going to become a tap dancer. Don't be afraid to have an ideal, of what you want in a man or a woman, however if your butt ugly your not going to get Miss America, unless you've got forty million dollars.

I once introduce a really nice guy to one of my closest girl friends. I thought they were very compatible. He used to come into my coffee shop. He was a very attractive, and fit man, he was in his late forties at the time, great sense of humor and I used to raise hell with him every day. My girl friend was a professional woman, quiet, sweet, sophisticated, a real lady, smart, attractive, and fun but maybe ten to fifteen lbs. heavy. I introduced them. They went out and got along great. But then he told me, he was really interested in a young girl, in her twenties that worked for me. She was my daughters age, very attractive and trim, tall. I said to him, what on earth makes you think this young girl would be attracted to you! I told the girl she was not interested. I told him, look in the mirror and be happy my girl friend wants you! He wound up dating my friend for about five years, they got along great, they took trips together. In the end he wound up about four hundred pounds. They broke up eventually but not over the weight, she had trouble with his grown children. The last time I saw him I could not believe it. He still thinks he looks great, she's the one that looks great now.

Reality, versus our fantasies, we can have both but don't confuse the two.

You need to have goals though, and they can be things that you always wanted to do but never had the time. Don't let your kids say, you must be in your second childhood. Some goals may seem unattainable at first, but if you persevere they can come to reality. If you always wanted to be on stage, join a theatre group in your town, most towns now have great ones. If you always wanted to go to school for something, look into it, their are a lot of adult schools now that will give you credit for life experiences. Travel the world that is my goal. There are things you can do if your fifty or eighty. Make a list. Keep the things, that you are now doing that you enjoy, or that are fun, or relaxation to you. Think about what you need in your life, or what you want in your life. Think about what you used to fantasize about, what you always wanted to be, or do. It doesn't matter if you think its ridiculous, if you always wanted to do it put it down. My kids thought I was mad when I went hot air ballooning. It was fantastic I would do it every week if I could afford it. I would own my own if I could afford it. Now divide the list into, daily, weekly, and annual activities. In other words you could go to the movies daily if you really loved them, you could go to the theatre weekly or monthly, you could take a trip annually or semiannually. Some of the activities can be relaxing, some can be physical. Going to the movies is relaxing, going bowling is physical they could both be weekly activities. If you always wanted to travel, put that down and think if you could go once a year or twice a year, where would you like to go. Its a lot cheaper than you may imagine. I go to Europe at least once a year for two weeks. A tour for two weeks, including four star hotels, or better, most meals and air and land travel is between $2,000.00 and $2,500.00 sometimes cheaper. A cruise for a week is even cheaper. If you plan it and put down a deposit you will go, and you will be so happy you did. From the time you make the arrangements it will be something you will look forward to. It will help with your diet, you'll be thinking of it when you go shopping. For the deposit you will need about one quarter of the total trip. You can buy insurance cheaply that will enable you to get your money back if something catastrophic happens, and you can't go. Or if something happens while you are over there and they have to send you back early. Last year I went to Spain, and while over there got an abscess tooth, I had already been traveling with friends for one week. They could not help me, I went to a hospital and a pharmacy but they could not do anything for me. The travel agency arranged for me to come back and I got back about half of the trip money once I was home. If you like to bowl, call the alley and see about joining a league, that will make you go weekly. Or a golf league or anything else you enjoy, a tennis club, go to the swimming pool at the Y. Take a computer course, or join a gym. Write a book, look into college courses, volunteer, at hospice, or schools, or hospitals, or nursing homes. If you would like to go back to college, look into financial aid, go to adult courses, once you put the money down you will go. Join that local theatre group, or your condo association. You'll meet lots of exciting new people. Performing on stage if you always wanted to do it, even in a small part or in the chorus is exciting and very fulfilling. Scan your local papers for what's going on in town. Our town is great for jazz clubs, and its mostly older people and its great fun. Look in the yellow pages, of your phone book, for what ever topic strikes your fancy. Just continue to increase your physical and mental stimulation. You will be "Hot", before you know it and wonder how the heck you got there!

Determination, Patience and Courage are the only things needed to improve any situation. And, if you want a situation changed badly enough, you will find these three things.

Anonymous

Chapter ten:

Spirituality

Another aspect of life that many of us neglect in the everyday hassle that has become our lives is Spirituality.

Now I am not talking, a specific religious denomination. I am talking Spirituality. In recent years, with all of the increased sex and violence, ruining our world, there also seems to be a small quiet rebirth of spirituality. There are lots of television shows now on , Miracles, Angels, after life, etc.

This year they have had a mini series on "Jesus", on "Mary" and many other religious topics. The country has re- thought such issues as prayers in schools and sporting events, the abortion issue and other laws that we had passed a few years ago banning or allowing them. They are actually doing studies in Hospitals and research on prayer curing people.

All of the scientific evidence is supporting the notion that prayer definitely helps cure people. Institutions such as the Catholic Church have come out this year and apologized for its attitude toward the Holocaust, and loosened its attitude toward gays. In our church we have gays and lesbians giving out communion. The English monarchy has just come out with a new decree, that from now on when a King or Queen is crowned they will not have to give allegiance to the Anglican Church, or to the protestant faith. They can now be any faith they want. King Henry VIII would turn over in his grave.

I personally am a Roman Catholic, I started out when I was young, as a seventh day Adventist, and then a Baptist. Many of my close family are one or the other. My in-laws by my first husband are all

Jehovah's. So I know a little about many religions, and while I choose to remain a Catholic, they are not always happy with me! But I don't care you see, because I feel God knows where I'm coming from. According to my church, I am a divorced woman, living in sin. I have a hard time with this, because, neither divorce was really my fault. I do not believe, that God wants us to remain alone, because we made a stupid decision when we were young and foolish. After my first divorce, however, this did bother me enough to go and get an annulment. Which is also foolish, but at the time it made me feel better. In the long run, all it did was allow me to remarry in the church the second time, so when he divorced me I could be right back in the same boat again.

Another big problem I have with the church is their stand on birth control, especially in countries like Africa or Haiti, where they tell the people they must not wear condoms, and they spread aids all over the place. Having said all this however, I do consider myself very spiritual and religious. I go to church, whether they want me or not every single Sunday. I also go to communion, and I say the Rosary every day and pray very often.

The church itself, is made up of man's laws, some are very old and dated laws and should be brought into this century. Such as not allowing priests to marry or allowing women to become priests. These are old outdated laws and should be changed. I am not here to change the church, however, I hope it will begin to use some common sense before its too late.

I believe, God knows where we are at, he knows our thoughts and reason. He knows we live in a very difficult world, and that our situations are not always of our own making. We have to deal with daily life, we need to feed ourselves, our families, we need to deal with violence and depravity every day. For this we need spirituality of some sort. We need to believe in a higher power, we need to believe that there is something better somewhere and that we will be rewarded or punished some day for our actions. Without the help of a spiritual presence in our daily life, it would be too difficult for us to continue.

When you feel down, depressed, over whelmed try it, ask what ever God you believe in to help you. We need to lean on him, and to give him our problems. He will help us with them. You will feel lighter, and more relaxed. When I pray my life goes 100% better, guaranteed!

I killed two birds with one stone, when I started remaking my physical self, I also started a regular schedule of daily prayer. While I am walking on my treadmill everyday, I say my rosary. It takes exactly a half a mile. For anyone who doesn't know what the rosary is, it is a series of prayers that Catholics say on counting beads. You can make up your own, regime if you are not Catholic or your religion doesn't have a daily prayer schedule of some sort. Or even use that time to simply reflect on something nice, or read something spiritual.

When I was a kid and going to parochial school the nuns always told us we should say the rosary every day, we thought they were nuts. But at this time in my life I needed a renewal, and a couple of personal minor miracles, caused me to do it that way. We started saying the rosary when my ex husband got cancer, he said it and so did I, and also both of my sisters. He got well, we continued with it. One day we told a girl who was not catholic and showed her how to do it. One rosary consists of a total of 50 Hail Mary's, in sets of ten, and after each ten, you say a small prayer called the Glory be to God, and an Our Father. while you are saying these prayers you concentrate on what they call mysteries of the rosary, which are stories from the bible. Well this girl, bought a pair of old rosary beads in an antique store. They were black, and so old that the medals between each ten beads were worn off so you couldn't see the pictures, and the Christ on the cross was also almost worn right off.

This girl used them to say the rosary every day however, and she did it for quite a while, but one day she told my sister and I she didn't think it was working for her. We told her just preserver and eventually she would get what she was praying for.

In the meantime, my sister and I were going to Rome, and my sister was taking her rosary beads to dip in the holy water at St Peters Basilica. The girl asked her to take her beads as well. We did, I took mine also. When we were in St. Peters, we could not find any holy water in the founts and we were disappointed. We asked someone and they said they "sold" holy water in the gift shop. That upset us, then suddenly as we walked around the church we saw, their was holy water in front of St Peters statue. We took the three pair of rosary beads and dipped them and wrapped the girls up in a paper towel. We did not unwrap it till we got home two weeks later, when we did, to our surprise, her beads were like new. The gold of the cross and the medals was restored and the faces back on the medals and Christ was back on the cross. Now you don't have to believe any of that, if someone told me that story, I would not believe it. It happened to me, and I know that. It was enough to keep me saying the rosary forever! So I say it as I do my half a mile every day. Then I put on the morning news and get down on the floor and do the rest of my exercises.

I have begun to pray a lot, and really concentrate on my praying, and just talking to God. It has helped me a great deal over the past two years. He always answers me. I have achieved everything I have wanted and then some. So you work out your own spiritual encounter, but do something even if its just, yoga or communing with nature. This came over my E mail the other day, it says it perfectly. A memo from God, The entire thing was very long but the first paragraph says it all. and I quote. I am God, today I will be handling all of your problems. Please remember that I do not need your help. If life happens to deliver to you a situation, that you cannot handle. Do not attempt to resolve it. Kindly put it in the SFGTD box . (Something for God to do). It will be addressed in my time, not yours. Once the matter is put into the box, do not hold onto it.

You may not get the answers you want but you will get the answer that is best for you.

When I first met Jim, my fiancée, I would go to church every Sunday. One of the very first things he said to me, was don't expect me to ever go to church with you. I told him of course not. He was from a catholic background but had never brought his children up in the church and had never gone himself. Not since he was a child. That was my thing and his soul was his own and I would never try to force anyone to do anything they did not feel. He felt no need to change. We had been going out maybe six months or so. One Sunday, out of a clear blue sky he told me he was going with me. I was very surprised and asked why, he just mumbled something about he had prayed for something and gotten it and had promised God he would go. Only once though! So he went. Slowly but surely as our relationship got stronger and longer he went more and more and now he goes every week. I have no idea what the deals he made with God are about I have never asked, but its apparent something is working for him, for him to change so drastically. He often asks me questions about the bible, and stories he hears in church he watches occasional bible stories on television.

Many times now we even leave the singles dances on Saturday night at 11:30 to get to midnight mass in Boston at St Anthonys. The bartender will even remind us, "Isn't it time for church you guys?"

Everything flow, and nothing stay. Herbalists (c.535-c.475 bc) Greek

Chapter Eleven:

Living Life for you!

Most of us mothers, (and some single father's who raised their children), by our very nature have lived most of our lives for other people. Whether you were married fifteen years, twenty five years, or thirty seven year, it was probably time totally dedicated to taking care of someone else. Intended or not, your time was consistently used caring for your kids, your mate, maybe even your siblings, parents, pets or neighbors and their kids.
    The list goes on. Someone else always came before you. When I was just sixteen, I had to take care of my stepfather as well as my three younger sisters and brother after our mother ran away from home.
    When I was eighteen, I got married to get out of the house, and exchanged caring for my step father and siblings for a husband and within a few short years seven children of my own. When I was twenty I had my first child, by twenty three I had four. During all the time I was raising them, I not only looked after them, but friends, family, other people's children, two dogs etc. I remembered the birthdays, and anniversary's of just about everyone I had ever met.
    Not just family but friends as well. I was always baking pies or cakes to bring to someone. Send over a card, have a little party etc. I would love it when they would ask, how do you remember everything? I took good care of myself, but I took better care of everyone else. I prided myself on having the cleanest, best dressed, best looking children in the town. How many birthday cakes did I bake? Did I ever get one back? My husband often called up at noon

to tell me he was bringing five or eight men home for supper at five. Usually clients from other countries. We entertained men from South America, Ireland, Holland and many other places. While I enjoyed it, having a three course meal on the table in a couple of hours for so many was not easy.

Of course the house had to be cleaned and the children scrubbed and out of the way. Or occupied for the evening. If it wasn't my husband it was the school. My children all went to Parochial school, and the mother superior was forever calling me for something or other. She called me a living saint for all the work I did for them. She knew she could depend on me to run the P.T.O and the fund raisers required to make money to keep the school afloat.

I usually made about 100 stuffed animals for their bazaar every year. I also always was the one to decorate the hall and to put on dances. The children of course had all kinds of needs from helping with homework, to going to ball games, being Brownie leader or Cub scout mom. I was constantly taxiing someone somewhere. Devoting time to their projects that had to be done the next day. You know the drill. We never had time for ourselves, by the end of every day you were exhausted. And of course you still had to give, if the old man was in the mood !

We worked all that time in anticipation of that distant time in the future, somewhere out there in another dimension, when it would be all over, and you could retire! One day they would all be gone and you would have that elusive time! We always had plans for that time. When the kids are grown, I will have time for my flowers. When the kids are grown, we will have a lawn. When the kids are grown, we'll make that bedroom into a sewing room. When the kids are grown, I will go back to school and finish my education. When the kids are grown, I will travel to exciting places.

Well, what are you waiting for !! Here's your chance. Stop feeling sorry for yourself. Make a plan. The time has come at long last. It may not be the way you pictured it, maybe your husband was in the plan with you, but believe me if you get over it, you will find you can have a much better time on your own. Don't waste any time feeling sorry for yourself, You have another 20 to 40 years of life left don't waste another minute. Plan like its going to be at least 40 so you need to take good care of yourself.

Now that your free, don't sit around missing the kids or your ex. Every body gets a little "empty nest" syndrome, but it's the way of the world. The little birds have to fly, and it they don't you are not a good parent. It's not good parenting having a child living at home at thirty years old. Enjoy your new freedom and make plans.

I remember the feeling, the very first time I walked into my new little apartment after my first divorce. I sat there in the quiet and the solitude. But I was not unhappy, I thought, I will never have to drive a kid to a function again! Yeahoo ! I will never have to cook for someone else again unless I invite company myself. I can do what I want when I want.

To prove the point sometimes I would get up in the middle of the night and go to the beach. I would tell people they could call me anytime of the day or night! It was wonderful, and overwhelming. I never once regretted my decision or wished for it to be back the way it was. You need a new lease on life. You've survived the worst, now the rewards. Don't jump right back into another marriage or any live in situation that's going to stifle your freedom again.

Learn to let other people do things for you for a change. I found that was one of the hardest things to adjust to. Letting people do things for you. My boyfriend would get up from the table and start to do the dishes, and I would say, Oh no, I'll get those. Or open a door for you, carry your packages, offer to do things. I had to learn to bite my tongue and let them do it. Just say, Thank you so much and sit back and enjoy it.

I have found many men love to cook, so let him. My son's love to cook, and their wives don't even think about butting it. We need to take a page from the younger generation of women, they expect to get waited on, and they do.

I never cook now. I let my children invite me to all the Holidays. I never entertain, unless it's a close girl friend or a gentleman. I deliberately bought a small condo and small kitchen table so I can't entertain. "Oh sorry I would love to have Christmas, but I just don't have the room!"

Besides it's their time. They need to develop their own holiday traditions. They enjoy entertaining as much as I used to. It would be most disappointing to them if they couldn't. Don't be critical of the way they do things. If they are going to develop their own traditions they need to be their own, not yours. Don't offer advice unless you are asked. It may not be your way but if the job gets done, leave it alone. Learn to shut up and think before you criticize, especially if it's your boyfriend or your child. Friends will generally tell you off. If you relax and just have conversation with them while they work, it will be an enjoyable experience for all. I look forward to spending one on one time with my adult children now just to chat and catch up on all the gossip.

An instance, of what I am talking about, the very first time I cooked a nice dinner for Jim, he complimented me on it, then got up from the table and started clearing the table and doing the dishes. I said, "Oh no hon I'll do that". He said, "Why"? You cooked the dinner didn't you? I can certainly help clean up. I realized if I hadn't let him do it, he would have felt he was not contributing to the relationship, and I backed off. Since then I have found out he can iron his own clothes, do the laundry, clean and cook as well as I can.

We women are too used to doing it all and it's not necessary. He does have a fantastic sense of humor and every day does something to crack me up! One night he cooked me a wonderful dinner, it was Ash Wednesday and as a catholic I told him in the morning that I had to have fish that night. I came home from work, and it was already. The table was beautifully set, he met me at the door with a lovely hug and kiss, walked me to the table and set me down. He turned around to take the fish out of the oven and I nearly died. He had cut the seat out of his pants and the cheeks of his ass were sticking through! He turned around with the pan of fish in his hands dead pan face, and said "what's the matter"? I was absolutely hysterical.

The meal was fantastic and he has cooked me many, many more

meals since then. His specialty and my favorite is a turkey dinner, he makes a fantastic turkey soup with the bones. He can also make a great pea soup another of my favorites. I can't even make soup!

Let people make you happy for a change. Jim keeps me on my toes with his great sense of humor, but as much as I love him, I do not ever want to get myself back into the situation that has preceded my past two divorces. I intend to make this a very long engagement. I feel unless it is somehow going to improve my life why get married again at this age?

My younger sister just got married this year after a twenty three year engagement. They raised three kids together, and had lots of ups and downs but never found the need to get married. They stayed together while many of our married friends broke up. Maybe there is a psychological feeling about being married. Maybe the marriage license makes people insecure or possessive. Remember if you choose to live together to get along with each other's kids that is an important point. The kids are already feeling a little insecure don't add to it.

Make sure you both contribute equally as your means allow to your living expenses and physically to what ever work needs doing. Discuss all these things before you decide to cohabitate. If one of you brings more in the way of money or investments to the arrangement cover your ass. Don't ever put your home or investments in the other persons name, unless you want to loose half of it. If you do weaken and get married have a pre-nuptial agreement or be sure you each have your own money in your own names in case it goes sour. You know from experience that can happen to the most wonderful of relationships. Can you afford to divide your assets down the middle again at your age? This is your new life, plan it around what you want not your significant other, and not your children. Be selfish for the first time in your life.

Chapter twelve:

How do I keep from making the same mistakes again?

So many, many people make the same mistakes, over and over again. I have two girlfriends I can think of right off the bat. One has been married five times, the other four times. They are both loving, attractive, caring, women. When they are married they do everything for their husbands. They always pick the same type man. One has been married to three alcoholics and is now going with another one. She hardly ever drinks.

The other one falls too hard too fast before she really knows the guy well enough. She lets him move in and does everything for him then realizes she has a leech and can't get rid of him. She finally does after months of fighting and all sorts of goings on. As soon as he is gone she does it again with another one. She just married a guy younger than her that she knew for one month. She has put him on her health insurance and she is trying to find him a job. We all know where this is going to end but she can't seem to see it!

Women who have been battered or abused always seem to pick the same types again and again unless they get a lot of counseling. But many of us who need counseling don't recognize that we need it unfortunately. I guess many of us have weaknesses from our childhood that makes us pick a certain type. We have to learn from our experiences. When you find yourself being attracted to someone, take some time by yourself and try to look at him objectively. Say to yourself, if this the type of guy I would want my daughter to wind up with? If not why not? If you can't see him objectively ask some real close friends who's opinion you can trust or members of you family and heed what they tell you.

Look objectively at other people's relationships what do you like about them, what do you not like? What kinds of things do you see happening in their relationships good or bad. Learn from them. Do not close your mind to what other people are telling you.

Pay attention, and even if you disagree, please give it some thought when you are by yourself, ask yourself honestly, is there any truth to what they are saying? We all know some "friends" can be jealous and will tell you bad things just to keep you from getting involved, but we all have really good, honest friends who will not do that. Listen to them. If eight out of ten people don't like him there has to be a reason.

Talk to your "adult" children, again teenagers usually don't want Mummy to get involved but older children usually want what's best for you. Once you've made them understand that you are going to date whether they like it or not they will be vocal about who they like and who they don't.

When I was going out with four guys at once, I liked them all. They were all very different and each had something different to offer, but my kids kept saying they liked Jimmy and eventually I realized what they saw and knew it was true. So, I am not saying to let other people pick your next beau, but if you know you are not good at it, give credence to their opinions.

Don't make excuses for bad behavior because your, "in love". The bad habits will still be there when the "love" has cooled down. Don't let your opinion be biased because your in love with love and are so anxious to find someone. When your tempted to make a quick or irrational decision, remember how long it took you to get out of your old situation.

Remember all the bad things in your marriage, is it worth it getting back into that? Both of the girlfriends I've mentioned are getting ready to get married again. I can see failure already because the guys that they picked are someone you should have a short fling with but not long term. If you have been out dating for a while, listen and pay attention to what your man does for you. Does he pay attention when you show him something in a store window you admire? If you make a comment, "I love that", when you're looking a magazine or watching television, does he make a mental note? Has he ever surprised you with something you thought was pretty? If you say I would love to do that, or go there, does he ever make plans? After going out for six months or more, does he have a clue as to what is your favorite color, or scent, or music? Does he surprise you with little notes, or cards or flowers or gifts for no reason.? Does he put thought into the gifts or just cover his ass with routine flowers or candy or something sexy he wants to see you in for his benefit?

Candy, flowers or a bottle of wine are nice and they are better than coming empty handed, but my favorite gifts from Jimmy were. A homemade apple pie, after I had commented in a restaurant that was my favorite dessert, (he even made the crust). A bacon press, which came in the mail after my commenting I wanted one. A bulletin board he put up in the bedroom, to tack little notes on stating why he loved me. Every time he came to my house he put another one on . A hot air balloon ride as a Christmas gift because I had once said I would love to do that one time!

These are gifts with meaning. It's not about the gift or the money spent, it's about listening! I want thoughtful gifts from someone I am considering a long term relationship with. Does he take you out on a long and lovely date before he starts getting sexual? Or is his favorite date, you cook dinner and we'll stay in and fool around?

Is he generous, does he have enough money but he's too cheap to spend it on you? One guy I dated took me to his house the first date, to show it off, it had to worth a million dollars easy, but he only took me to a coffee shop to eat and then wanted to go back to his house to fool around. I dated him a few times, but it never changed, so I dropped him quick. I started talking to a couple of other girls who knew him and found out the same thing happened with them, now three years later he can't get a date with anybody!

Rich doesn't mean anything if they keep it to themselves. A poor man who shares what he has is better. When you discover something about your man that you don't like, don't overlook it. It won't get better. For instance, at the beginning of my relationship with my second husband, he would fly into a rage over nothing and swear at me and call me all kinds of names. I was so crazy about him that I made excuses for his behavior. He would always come back and apologize and tell me how much he loved me. Sixteen years later I finally realized I had been verbally abuses for years. It never got any better, my life was one of constant ups and downs. One minute he would be making over me and loving me and the next yelling cursing and swearing at me. It was very stressful and I bounced back and forth from loving to hating him all the time.

A man who truly loves you will want to please you as much as he can. He will not want to abuse you, mentally, verbally or physically. His state of mind is no excuse. While there is no absolute way to be sure that the man you are dating is marriage, or long term relationship material, time is the best measuring stick. He can't be on his best behavior for years. That is why it is not a good idea to jump into a live-in situation in a big hurry. Give it a lot of time and pay attention to the signs. I have been going out with Jim for four years now. There are times when his stubbornness, (which is his only really bad trait), drives me nuts! Yet he is so sweet and considerate the rest of the time, that it is hard to believe that he can be so narrow minded at these stubborn times.

I have told you of the wonderful things he has done else where in this book. Most of the time he thinks I am the most wonderful woman that has ever lived. What is more, he believes that and convinces me of that. He goes out of his way every day to tell me in new and exciting ways that he loves me. For instance, one day I came home from work to find a note on the table from Jim telling me how wonderful I was it went on and on, he said, "it was time the world knew how wonderful I was". He had traveled fifty miles away to a mall in Nashua to put my name in a contest on "The Hollywood Squares".

The following day he cleaned the kitchen from top to bottom. It sparkled, but the next day I could not find my dish sponge. I asked him about it, he had used it to clean the kitchen and then had thrown it away. I explained to him that I kept sponges under the sink for such cleaning jobs, but that the sponge he threw away was just for dishes. That afternoon when I came out of work for lunch and got in my car, there was a tremendous bag tied up with a bow. Inside there were all sorts of funny shaped sponges.

When a man takes time to do these kinds of things, you know he is really trying. He is doing everything in his power to please you. His most endearing trait to me, is that he is not possessive. If he doesn't feel like going dancing or on a trip I want to go on, he has no problem with me going by myself with my girl friends. He would never ever tell me I couldn't go. If I had lunch with a male friend that I had known for a long time, he would have no problem with it. One night that I was at the Grog for instance dancing with my girl friend I met a new young fellow, he was actually there with his girl friend, but he liked me right away and we got into conversation. The following day he came by where I worked to take me to lunch. I let him know I had a boy friend and that I was not interested in anything but being friends. That night I told my boyfriend about this young 34 year old guy coming by work and taking me to lunch. All Jim said was, "Good going" and hi-fived me. That's the way he is, he knows I love him and would never be unfaithful, I love having a steady companion and yet being able to be myself and do what I want.

If a man meets you more than half way, if he shares his time and money with you, if he is not jealous or possessive, if he doesn't try to change you, or tell you how to dress, If he tries to make friends with you friends and family, if he wants you to go to his family get togethers and introduces you to his kids. Then you know he is a keeper.

Chapter thirteen: Class!!

Fred Astaire, Ivanna Trump, Prince Charles

If you are going to be out there on your own, there are several attributes you may want to develop, or try to develop. It will give you a "Mistique" you were lacking. You will have less problems, and you won't be singled out for ridicule or be taken advantage of. These attributes can help you to become popular. They are things that usually come naturally, you generally either have them or you don't . You may already have them, but if I describe them to you you will know. Or you can ask your friends if they feel you have them. If you don't have them, I think it is possible to develop them with a little work. The first one is "Class". Class is a quality that sets you apart
from other people in the room who don't have it. It's hard to define, yet you know when people have it. For example if you compare, Marilyn Monroe with Lauren Bacall. Marilyn is gorgeous but Lauren has class. Both women were famous, popular, beautiful, sexy but Bacall had class, Marilyn did not. Class is a combination of coolness, aloofness, good manners, regal appearance, friendliness, quality, and patience. The main words I think are Cool and Quality. It don't so much have to do with beauty or the way you dress as it does with the image you portray. The way you conduct yourself, the way you put your clothes together, quality not quantity. It doesn't matter so much what size you are, how attractive you are, if your rich or poor, but what you do with it. You may be able to pick out instantly a person with class when they enter a room. Or you may need to know someone for a long time to sense that they have it. The way a person moves, sits, eats or handles a precarious situation. Let me try to give

you some examples as it is so hard to define.

Lets say you are in Central Park. You see two street people picking through the trash to find something to eat or wear. The first one eats with his fingers, right out of the containers at the trash barrel continuing his search as he eats. The other one puts his treasures in a plastic bag, stopping to take a scarf out of the trash, which he puts around his neck in a jaunty manner. Then he takes his delicacies under a tree, lays them out neatly and eats with a much treasured plastic fork and wipes his face with a bit of paper napkin. Which one very obviously has class, despite his sorry state in life? He is hanging on to a vestige of class that is important to him. He is retaining his dignity about doing the best he can with what he has.

The first man has allowed himself to turn into an animal as a result of his bad time. Another less dramatic example is, it's a stormy night and there is a big formal party. The guests are arriving and the women as usual are whining about their hair and stepping in water in their delicate shoes etc. All night long they are overly concerned about how they look and continue to whine about it. One lady comes in, she is also wet her hair do is ruined and dripping. However, she comes in smiling and greeting everyone, she also comments about the weather and her appearance but does it in a laughing and jovial manner. She takes a towel and pats herself as dry as she can, slicks her hair back and does not mention the weather or her appearance again all night. She continues enjoying herself and greeting everyone in her gracious manner. Which one has class, which one would you prefer to spend the evening with? If you have class you always try to act in a "regal" manner, with a quiet coolness and humor about everything. You do not say hateful things about anyone, you try to be nice to everyone equally. You may dress elegantly, simply or eccentrically, but always with a certain flair.

An ascot, a strategically placed scarf, pin or flower. A handkerchief in a man's suit pocket, or a flower in his lapel. A cocky tip of the hat, something that shows your individuality and sets you apart from the crowd. God forbid that you smoke, but if your one of those that just can't quit, use a holder, its classy and it will help filter the nicotine. In your behavior, you can show class in the way you handle a disagreement or a dispute.

You can be the person who tries to see everyone's point of view, and point out the good points to the confronting party. Every opinion has some good points. You can have strong opinion's, but be willing to hear the other side and try to understand their reasoning for it. The most important thing in a conflict is always stick to the point of the disagreement don't turn it personal. If it's a conflict between you and someone else, try to take the high road in resolving the issue. Be the bigger man, as they say. Don't stoop to cursing and violence to make a point unless there is no other solution.

Sometimes you can disarm the other person, if he is yelling and cursing to say quietly to him or her, "you don't need to curse", or something kidding like, " Do you kiss your baby with that mouth?" This does not mean that if you are a little loud and fun loving that you can't have class. If your loudness is connected to the fun you are having, and you are the center of attention, as long as everyone is comfortable and you are including everyone in the fun you can still do it with class.

You can teach people how to make light of a tense situation with your cool attitude. You can make fun of a bad situation like the girl in the rain did. For instance sometimes at the singles they will serve messy finger foods like fried chicken. We don't usually eat before we go, because we know they are going to feed us. Some of the girls won't eat if it's something messy, even though they are starving. God forbid they mess up their makeup or look unattractive eating with their fingers. One night I took a good sized plate of chicken, I was seated at a round bar so their were lots of guys right across from me. I ate it as ladylike as I could, but my fingers were still all messy when I got through. So I proceeded to lick my fingers very seductively, while giving the eye to the guys across the bar. They went nuts!

Now I'm sure I would get an argument about that being classy, but the point is when you are in an uncomfortable situation, make fun. For a while after that every time we had chicken we would make a game out of who could do it the most seductively. Class doesn't swear, whine or bitch unnecessarily. Class does not drink from a beer bottle, get a champagne glass, your beer will look beautiful in a champagne flute. Never leave your house without makeup, or with your hair in rollers or not done if you have to go somewhere before you have time to do your hair, wear a hat. Class never dances in your stocking feet, bring a pair of flat shoes in your car or purse. You can get those flat ballet slippers that will fit in your purse or go out to your car and change if you have to. If you plan a picnic, pack a cloth tablecloth and wine glasses, even if they are plastic wine glasses, have real silverware and cloth napkins. Have fresh flowers and candles or aroma around your apartment. Remember to always act with sophistication, whether in jeans or in satin you will always have class.

Chapter fourteen:

Charm! Shirley Temple, Carey Grant, Bill Clinton & Rosie O'Donnell

Charm goes hand in hand with class, but it's not the same thing. For instance Rosie has oodles of charm but is lacking in class. Bill, also. You can have charm without class, and class without charm. If you can develop both you have to be a winner.

Charm is also hard to define. It can be a twinkle in your eye, or a dimple in your cheek. Charm can be an inanimate object, like a lace collar or a picture hat. It can be a bit of flirting, a lilt of laughter, a wink of an eye, a raised shoulder, a toss of the head, a touch, or a cute cowlick . Lots of things can be charming, lots of things can make us charming. A person can be charming, a picture can be charming, a tiny church, or a whole town can be charming, a room, a scene.

I just came back from Bavaria where everything is charming. Even the cows with bells on their hand embroidered collars, and flowers on their horns were charming ! Some people are born charming, but if you are not that fortunate you can develop charm. It's something that intoxicates people and draws them to you. It could be a mannerism, a way that you do things, that no one else does, a cute habit that is unique to you. Unlike class you can be charming while being totally obnoxious. You can be charming swearing, or loud or crass. It's the way you come across.

For instance, I used to tend bar in a quaint little pub up on Lake Winnipisaukee. An old lady, used to come to sit at my bar. She had to be eighty or more, she was a tiny little thing and had to climb up on the stool. She looked like the original old lady from that poem, "When I grow old, I shall wear Purple". She would talk and tell stories and curse and swear like a dock worker and smoke cigarettes from a very long holder. She dressed very eccentrically, usually a wild hat. She was charming as hell and we never tired of her. Now a twenty year old doing the same thing would not be as charming. She was funny and I have to say she had a lot of class as well. I adored her.

Many older men are very charming, they have developed over the years, a way about them, that is very gracious and appealing. They may kiss your hand, or look directly into your eyes and tell you how lovely or absolutely marvelous you are. It could be a lot of BS. but its very charming. You love it even though you know its probably not true. Think about what intrigues you about other people. What do you consider charming?

Many of the women in the singles scene get very upset with men who tell them lies and lead them on. I find these men charming and love to raise hell with them. Once you let them know your on to them they won't lie anymore. Or you simply let them know you don't believe one word they say but you like them anyway. They can become your biggest allies. These guys you make up a bigger story and tell them. They won't know what to make of you, but you can enjoy each other. Sometimes charm is teasing and mischievous. Charm can be an adjective or a verb. You can turn on the charm. You can be charming. A teapot can be charming. It covers everything. So begin by smiling, laughing out loud, be a good sport, and try to develop just a little charm. The very first thing that attracted me to my fiancée, was the big dimples in his cheeks and his fantastic smile. The minute I commented on his dimples, he really worked it. He also has a mischievous look in his eye that warns of a very dry sense of humor. He hooked me, he is one of the most charming men I know.

Chapter fifteen:

Don't be too easy!

No matter how much they say the world has changed, there is still always going to be a double standard for behavior between men and women. A man can have twelve women all going at the same time and he's a cool popular guy. All the other men will, "Hi five" him all over the place, and envy him. If a woman does the same, she's a slut. There isn't a word I know of that can be used to describe a male slut. Don't let that bother you too much, you just have to be careful how you conduct yourself.

If you go to singles clubs, you will see many women being aggressive, and the men claim they like it. If you ask the men standing around the dance floor why they are not approaching the women, or asking them to dance they will say, why don't they ask us to dance? Times have changed you know. We don't want to be embarrassed by having them turn us down. These same men however will talk about you if they see you being too loose or aggressive.

If you see a man you are interested in you have to be aggressive either in a subtle or more active way. If you don't want to be asked to dance all night by men you are not interested in, you have to let the ones know that you are interested in. Your best moves are pick out who you are attracted to early, before another woman makes a move on him. Smile start a conversation. Most of the guys are easy, if a fairly attractive woman asks them to dance, or just start a conversation, he will stay with her all night. Most men are afraid of rejection. They only get aggressive when they have had a few drinks and it's after eleven p.m. and they want someone to take home. Then they will hit on anybody. By that time you want to be with someone you picked out, or get out of there. At that time of night the guys wander around half in the bag talking to anyone.

Once you've met a man you like, it's hard to ride the fence between being your own woman and being considered easy. Especially if you want to eventually be monogamous with someone but don't want to get remarried. In order to find Mr. Right, you have to date a lot of men. In order to date a lot of men, you have to become popular. How do you do that without getting a bad reputation? You have to start by being friendly with everyone, even the geeks. If the handsome ones see you being friendly, laughing with men, and women. They will approach you.

You want to be just as friendly with women as men. If the women don't like you they can be brutal, and they will be the ones to ruin your reputation. You can be good friends with the less popular men, dance with them, joke with them. Just let them know right up front that is all you are looking for. They will become your allies. If they ask you out because they misread your friendship, and you don't want to go out with them. Let them down gently while retaining the friendship.

There are many ways to do this, such as, I would love to have coffee with you but I am only looking for a friend not a sexual partner. This will usually make them back off. They are generally looking for a sexual partner, but they will still talk to you when you are at the clubs. Or, say I would love to but I am already dating a couple of men, so I am not looking for another boyfriend, just a friend.

There are lots of ways to discourage an unwelcome suitor, find out what they are looking for in a woman and be the opposite. One very unattractive man who followed me around for weeks got completely turned off when he found out I lived a good sixty miles from where he lived. He was cute, he told me I really like you but you live too far away. I feigned disappointment. He still talks to me but doesn't pursue me anymore. One of my favorite lines when I was dating several men at one time was, "sorry I would love to go out with you, but my program is full, I have a guy for every day in the week, I can't possibly fit another guy into my schedule". For weeks they would continue to ask me. Do you have room yet? Let me know when you have an opening. They would walk around telling other people, I can't believe she's dating seven guys!

As long as you are not insulting to them, you can turn a guy down and still stay good friends. Pick the guys you want to date that are honorable, that won't be talking behind your back. You can tell by the questions you ask when you first meet them. Ask them questions about a previous girlfriend or someone at the singles you know they have dated. If they start saying nasty things about her, or calling her names, a bitch, a slut, anything, you know that is how they will talk about you when you stop seeing them.

All the guys I dated, had class, they never said anything bad about another woman, they were very closed mouthed about everything. The other thing is be totally honest from day one, but don't tell them too much. If you are dating other guys let them know that, but don't ever tell details. Chances are you will run into the other guys at the singles and you don't want to have to duck out or be afraid to introduce the two guys to one another if it becomes necessary, which it may if they both come over to you at the same time.

I have a rule if you did not pay my way in, I am not with you. I owe you nothing. The first time any of them asked me out, I always told them I was dating other guys and if they had a problem with that we would not go out. I would tell them I am not interested in marriage, but I might be interested in a relationship down the road. They all accepted that, and would usually say the same thing to me.

The girls that I know that got a bad rep for dating more than one guy, made the mistake of letting them think they were the only one in their life at the time. If both guys showed up at the same place they went out the back door! One particular girl that I know did that so many times that none of the guys would go out with her again and they all talk about her. I don't even see her around anymore, I think she made it impossible for her to keep coming. For a time she was one of the most popular girls around. Attractive blonde, great figure, she had half the guys in the place drooling all over her. She dated, and slept with one after the other, but always let them think they were her only boyfriend. They would show up at the same place and get into a fight over her. I dated more men at one time than she ever did, but I let them all know that.

I was never possessive, I let them do as they pleased, I did the same. When I eventually broke up with all of them, they were disappointed, but I let them know it was not personal. We are all still good friends. I know if I was single again tomorrow they would ask me out again. I am not flattering myself but I know it's true. So, be very friendly and full of hell with everyone.

Be helpful, introduce friends to each other. Build a network of friends you can depend on. Let people hear you laughing out loud at someone's jokes. Tell a few yourself. Be a good listener, look people in the eye. Be interested in everyone and everything. Be particular with the men you want to date.

From the first moment you meet them, make every question informative to you. Ask questions in such a way as to get information about them. "What's your name?", "Is this your first time here"?, "Where else do you go to meet people"? The answers to this questions are telling you, if he goes out often, is he promiscuous. "What do you do for work?" "Do you come from around here?" Then if that is going well, get into, "have you been alone for long"? By now you will know what he does, where he lives, and if he is divorced, widowed, separated or always single and how long.

They will usually add how long their last relationship was, like they may say "I am just coming off a three year relationship. This information is important in making judgments about sex. If a man says, "I am coming off a five year relationship", we just broke up. Or my wife died last year this is my first time out. You have a pretty good idea he has not been with a lot of women.

On the other hand, if he is fairly aggressive with you and says, "Yea I come here often, I also go to Vincent's on Thursday and the Palace on Tuesdays, you have a pretty good idea he is probably promiscuous if given the chance. You may still wish to pursue a relationship with him but you will be well advised to use protection for sexual encounters. You should do that anyway, but if making judgments about these things all this has to be considered, and I am giving you ideas of how to get this information without direct questions that they may find offensive.

When a man tells you he has been divorced for ten years and has been coming to the singles three times a week since then, you have a pretty good idea he is not looking for a life partner. Make every question be informative to you. Don't ask questions just to talk and not pay attention to the answers. Everything they say tells you something about them, and if the next morning you can't remember anything about them you did not do a good job.

The most important thing, should be getting to know him. Many people talk just to be talking they are swept up in the feelings of the moment, they are reacting to the chemistry, touch and sight, rather than listen. Guard against that, this information can be invaluable to you later on. If you feel tempted to take him home for some much needed sex, fight the feeling. Try to hold out for a date, but we are only human, if you give in use a condom. Don't feel that because you had sex, that he owes you something or that it means anything other than sex. Not that its not possible for it to develop into more, but its not usually the case. If you are as nonchalant about it as a man would be, and he sees that he may well come back for more. But a guy doesn't want to think that he has to marry you because you had one night of passion, and some women make him feel that way.

Men do not want to be made to feel guilty or that they owe you something because they had sex with you. If you really want a relationship, try to hold off, make him take you out first, get to know him better. If he continues to pursue you after you've turned him down, he is interested. If he doesn't you'll know that's all he is after. Having sex right away will not absolutely keep him from pursuing you, but like everything else you need to handle it properly. For instance lay your cards on the table, with humor, "I'm sorry I attacked you, I just couldn't help myself you are so attractive". "I hope it will not stop you from calling me again". "I promise I'll try to control myself the next time". goes a very long way at making a guy feel great and letting him know you are interested.

If all else fails use humor, it gets me through so many tight spots. Another time a guy traveled over sixty miles to take me out. The chemistry between us the first time was very strong, and I knew before the evening was over we would be in bed. I was looking forward to a nice long evening and dinner and getting to know him. When he came to the door, we immediately started kissing hello, but the kisses were getting very hot. So I suggested we have sex right then and there before we went out and get it out of the way so it wouldn't interfere with the rest of our evening.

He thought it was the coolest thing he had ever heard it worked our evening was very easy going afterwards. We dated for more than six months. He still gets a kick out of it.

When you first meet a man and are trying to get information out of him, you need to be subtle, this bares repeating. Ask so they won't recognize that you are being nosey. Don't fire direct questions at them like a machine gun. "What's your name, how old are you, are you married, divorced, have a good job, any kids etc. etc.

Instead ask a question, pause listen to the answer comment on it. Then ask another question. Word your questions in such a way that you cover a lot of territory with one question, such as. Do you come here often? This will open up the whole series of questions. They might say, no this is my first time, I just got a divorce last month. Your next question then can be, "were you married a long time?" "Do you have any children?" (Your comments between questions, can be complimentary to him.) For instance, what's your name?…Craig.. oh I love that. "Hi Craig", (in your sexiest voice). Why would any woman divorce a gorgeous man like you?

Very often questions asked in jest or in a humorous way will still bring forth an honest answer. "Oh the divorce wasn't all her fault, I was a jerk". Or I often kidding around will say to a guy when he asks me out, "Sorry I need to see your portfolio first". Even though this is a kidding around kind of statement it often invokes an honest response. "Oh my portfolio is pretty good", or "I'm afraid I lost a few thousand dollars in last years crash".

Or the opposite, "Huh, I don't have a portfolio, but I have a pretty good job". There are all sorts of ways to get information out of him without him even knowing it. Oh you poor man, I bet you could use a home cooked meal. What do you do for a living? Oh that sounds so interesting, tell me more. Do you have to travel far to go to work? That question will generally get you the answer to both where he lives and what he does.

Be discrete and careful, men don't like nosey women, but they love to brag. You have to make it sound like casual conversation, not the third degree. Teasing and humor will go along way. Don't ask personal questions about his divorce or his ex. They will volunteer that.

Some women are so direct or say things in such a way the man will immediately walk away. I have actually heard women start a conversation with a man with, "So you gonna buy me a drink?", "No what are you a cheapskate?" Or something like, "So, what's your story"? They sound so confrontational the guy is speechless. then when he walks off they'll say, what a jerk. If you get the correct information up front it can help you to determine who you can have an intimate relationship with and who you can't.

When I was dating a lot of guys all the same time, I was probably having sex with four or five of them. I did not use a condom, which is foolish, but I didn't. I was pretty certain that none of them was seeing anyone else. Because in getting to know them they inadvertently told me, when their last long term relationship was and when they had last had sex. On the other hand a couple of others I was dating I could tell right away that they were dating numerous women and I did not have sex with them. Knock wood, I was lucky I never ever had even a yeast infection. Likewise I never had a bad reputation, because I did not leave a place with a guy, I did not make out on the dance floor and I did not make out in cars in the parking lot.

A lot of people would say I am naïve that you can never be sure of what a guy is doing and they are basically right. However, I have a different relationship with most guys than most girls. I am a friend,

I don't get shocked, I tell them the truth and expect the same. I've gone out with groups of guys as one of the gang. I am content that I got the correct information and made the right judgments for me. The ideal situation of course is to use protection all of the time. The ideal situation is to have one partner, which I have now, but to get to that point takes a lot of doing.

You do the right thing for you, don't take chances. What is an ideal situation is not always easy in real life. You meet someone, you have feelings, you have needs, you sometimes take chances. You shouldn't but you do, be as informed and as honest as you can. I am not responsible for you, only you are. If you feel confident that the men you are dating are safe, and that they are discrete in what they talk about with other people, you can have several relationships going at once with no worries about your reputation. In the beginning, however as hard as it is, hold out for a while, from having that first sexual encounter. Kissing and touching can go a long way for a while.

One hard fast rule, never, never go home with a guy from a bar or club the first night you meet him. Never go out to the car with him, when you have just met him to make out. A good night kiss and a hug are o.k. but no heavy petting.

There are several reasons for this, and I have heard the people talk when a girl does this. The obvious reason, if he really likes you he will call. If he is looking for a one night stand, the second you say no he will move on to someone else, and you will be very glad you didn't have sex with him. If he asks for your number and you like him, give it to him, but then forget that you gave it to him, and don't attack him when he comes in next week if he didn't call. If he likes you he will call, but on his own time not yours.

To a girl when a guy gets her number she thinks he will call the next day. To a guy when he takes your number, even if he likes you, it means he will call you sometime when he's looking for a date. Guys don't call to chit chat like girls do. They only call for a reason. Don't pursue him, if he doesn't call good riddance. Your persistence will only make him sure he was right not to call you. When he calls make him take you out, don't invite him over. Make him take you to dinner or a movie. You know if you invite him over, or if you go to his place its just for sex. Let him work and pay for it. Try to hold off till the next date or longer. Sometimes you can kid your way out of it. "I would love to have sex with you, but I have a three date rule", you know for sure your going to get that third date"! Probably even three times in the same week. This lets him know you are interested and not a prude but that you do have rules and standards.

By the third date you should know if this is a relationship you want to pursue further. If you don't and you don't want to have sex with him just cancel the third date. Or it could be the fourth, fifth or sixth date, make your own rules.

You could also tell a lie, I would love to have sex with you but it's the wrong time of the month. The trouble is not too many guys are discouraged by that. I don't even like to have a guy walk me to my car. It's safer and a very polite and caring gesture, but all the people who see you leave assume something is going on. When one of my male friends wants to walk me to my car, I make them go right back in the place afterwards so they can see he did not leave with me.

The other solution is have a couple of girlfriends walk you out. Many men walk you to your care on the pretext of being polite, but then try to jump you when you get there. I get in my car quickly, tell them no, lock the door, and finish saying good night through a crack in the window. If people are leaving and they see you making out inside or outside of the car, it quickly leads to a bad reputation. I have heard men describe women as, "She's a parking lot job". I never want to be one of those. That usually intimates that she will give you, "head" or a "blow-job" in the parking lot. No one wants that reputation.

So bottom line, do what you feel, think about it, think about the ramifications of your actions. Women are in command now, much more than they used to be, but we are still held to a higher standard then men.

It is possible however, to date half the guys at the singles club, and still do it with class and style. Lastly do not ever, not go there, because you just broke up with someone and he might be there. Let him stay home, not you. Don't let a man drive you away from your favorite place to go, because you are not dating anymore. Don't be mean to an ex or talk bad about him. Always stay friendly.

Chapter sixteen:

Love, Love, Love

My favorite passage from the bible is the one on love. Although it has been done to death at every wedding there is, which ultimately turn into ugly divorces, I still love it. If people would only listen to the words and take them to heart, the world would be a better place, because all the truth of love is here.
Love is patient, love is kind. Love is not jealous. It does not put on airs, it is not snobbish. Love is never rude! It is not self seeking, it is not prone to anger, neither does it brood over injuries. Love does not rejoice in what is wrong but rejoices in the truth. There is no limit to loves forbearance, to its trust, its hopes, its power to endure. Love never fails. Prophecies will cease, tongues will be silent, knowledge will pass away. Our knowledge is imperfect, and our prophesying is imperfect. When the perfect comes, the imperfect will pass away. When I was a child, I used to talk like a child, think like a child, reason like a child. When I became a man, I put away childish ways, Now we see indistinctly, as in a mirror. Then we shall see face to face. My knowledge is imperfect now, then I shall know even as I am known. There are in the end three things that last: Faith, Hope and Love and the greatest of these is Love!!
Love has always been a most indefinable emotion. That is why I include this Biblical explanation. God's definition is as good as it gets. Do you think any relationship would ever go awry if we honestly lived these words? No way but we are human, and to hold to this to the letter we would have to be saints. We humans often confuse emotions with love. Most people say love is love. there are many

different kinds of love to be sure. There are many kinds of emotions that we confuse with love, that are not love at all. There are also many kinds of love, or we manifest it in many ways. The love we feel for our child is different than the love we feel for our spouse. You love your cousin, your mother, your friends, your partner, your pet all in different ways, yet they are all forms of love. We say we love inanimate objects, I love my car, that dress in the window, I love my work, my hobby, my music, my country, your hair style, that furniture, we really mean we like it a lot but we don't love it. It's a stronger version of like, I love your gown. Sounds way more sincere than I like your gown, but we don't really love it.

It is no wonder that our feelings are confused when we are looking for a new love, because not only are our like feelings in there but they are all mixed up with our lust feelings. You would think after living 50 or 60 years we would have figured it out by now! How can we still be confused about love. I think the more love affairs we have the more confused we get, because if we can be fooled that many times can we trust our emotions?

There are many passions that we confuse with love, there are many depths of love. Here is where we must be cautious, sometimes the deepest passions are not the longest lasting. We must be aware of this when we are single and making new acquaintances. Otherwise you can easily be, "in love", every day. The trouble with this deep passion is it sometimes dies as quickly as it comes, and we could be walking around in misery all the time. We have to know it for what it is and deal with it. Don't be in a hurry to fall in love, take a new relationship slowly. Try not to think of it in a "love" sense think of it as a new friendship only. Forbidden love is usually the most intense, and the most fleeting. That is why your teenager will defy your orders to stay away from a boy or girl that you have forbidden them to see.

How can it be bad when it feels so good! The same with you, a strong handsome man, coming on strong, or a one night stand from someone who is your dream man can sweep you off your feet. Then drop like a rock, when he doesn't call you again. You can go over the fantastic sex, the unbelievable feelings in your head over and over and it can drive you to do stupid things. Drive by his house, dress up in something unbelievably sexy and go see him, call him, buy him presents, stupid things to get him to notice, when even if he does it will just be another wild but fleeting night.

Nothing is more disappointing or discouraging or takes more out of you. It can send you back into your shell with more feelings of inadequacy. Don't fall for it as tempting as it is. "Get thee behind me Satan". It's hard but hold out for a real date. When you have it, listen to everything he says, but until you know him, take everything he says with a grain of salt. Every man even the good ones, is going to say what he thinks you want to hear.

You have to get by that, first trying to impress you time, and get into the legitimate real and honest feelings time. It's easy to fall in love, especially if you are vulnerable, on the rebound, or haven't had anyone in a long time. Everyone wants to love and be loved. Everyone wants to be complimented. It's the most wonderful thing in the world to have someone tell you, you are the most wonderful, or beautiful woman he has ever met. That you are beautiful, witty, sexy, intelligent and on and on. Men looking for a new relationship or a new mate, know that. They know women are suckers for compliments and gifts.

Sometimes its genuine, but sometimes its just a line, you have to learn to know the difference to keep from being hurt. You need to step back, and hear it as if it were coming from a stranger, or if you heard someone say that to another girl, is it believable? Is it sincere, do his actions back up his words? Does he treat you as if you are the most important person in the world? All the time or just when he wants something? Does he respect you? Does he help you, is he polite? My boyfriend always unlocks the door for me, but steps back and waits for me to go first even if he is loaded down with packages.

I noticed that first thing. At the moment they are complimenting you they may feel that way for the moment, but is it long lasting or is it said to get a reaction? Be cautious take time, build the relationship gradually. My fiancée tells me, the first woman he went home with after two years of celibacy after his divorce, he told he loved her. He hardly knew her, but in the intensity of the moment, as he was having his much needed release, he blurted out, "I love you!" Needless to say he was embarrassed and the girl knew he didn't mean it, but some women would take it to heart. They would be telling their friends, he loves me, he told me so.

Try to develop friendships before you let your heart go. You will generally find the most lasting relationship is the one that develops more slowly. It may even be a relationship that started as a friendship and gradually blossomed into love. It may have even happened so slowly it surprised you, and you wonder when it changed. The first person that got you "hot", with a touch or smile, but didn't call you after the one night stand may be doing that with several other women.

Taking it all very lightly and never falling in love. I can tell you how to land him, but he will never make you happy. You'll always be waiting for another more exciting woman to come along and take him away from you. That type of man, becomes interested in you, when you are elusive, and ignore him. He has so much ego, he can't believe you would ignore him and he will pursue you till he catches you and then move on. He has so many different women he can have with a snap of his fingers, that if you show disinterest, he becomes interested. You become a challenge to him, but there is always a bigger challenge, a prettier, younger, richer, sexier, whatever one. So the only way to hold a man like that is to play the same game, but its very tiring.

Continuing to feign interest in another man until he gets jealous and comes back to you. Using him in the same way he uses you, showing lots of other men attention in front of him, and not falling head over heels in love with him. I'm sure you know many couples who play this game, it can be tedious and unfulfilling. It's not a good permanent situation. Forbidden love, feels good at the moment, but it's not long lasting. The most satisfying love is the quiet love that grows day by day. It builds and becomes a part of you. It's understood and grows by giving and receiving each day. You must not take it for granted, you have to keep working on it. Nurturing it. In the end it will be worth it. You will be happy and satisfied and you will have found as true a love as you can find on this earth.

Chapter seventeen:

Who already has it? "Hot, Hot, Hot" !!

I am not setting myself up as judge and jury, but I think their are certain people, both famous and not so famous, that to me exemplify the word in it's purest form. The people that I admire most, is as follows: I will start with some famous people that we all know so that you can understand what I am talking about. Then I will tell you about some people in my world that I admire and the reasons that I do.

The first famous woman I admire is Hilary Clinton. Now may I say I do not like her, there is no reason for that other than she just rubs me the wrong way. I don't know her but my perception of her, causes me to dislike her. I still admire the way she handles herself. In her personal life, her husband, (whom I love), mad a complete fool of himself. It was totally stupid, but it was a man thing. Hilary stayed cool, she acted with dignity, grace and candor. She did not break up her home or marriage. She led her own life, and is now a Senator and making a name for herself. She continues to be a great mother and supportive wife. She is constantly remaking herself, she is never boring. I am sure Bill is paying on some level for what he did to her, but its not out in public. She is a winner.

The second famous woman I admire is Tina Turner: Tina is my kind of woman, I like her both personally and publicly. She not only overcame a terribly abusive relationship, she continued with her career, without Ike and is more popular than she ever was. More exciting, more attractive, more dynamic. Now in the middle of her life she says she is retiring to spend her life helping out other women, being more spiritual, and enjoying the rest of her life with her younger beau. I envy her and admire her for many things. She looks terrific, much more attractive than she was when she was younger. She has a much younger lover, because men her age do not have the energy level she has. She makes friends and values them. I hope she will be with us many many more years, even if she retires.

For men that I admire, it is hard to find one and stick to, because admirable men have a way of eventually "fucking up" and ruining their status! Excuse my French but no other word adequately describes it. For a long time, I admired Donald Trump, I read his biography, I followed his and Ivanna's exploits. I didn't even change my mind when they got divorced because I knew his first love was business and I didn't expect him to stay married. Then he married that hard bodied young model and I began to change my mind toward him, had a baby with her first, I didn't like that. The final stupid thing he did was when he talked about running for the presidency but was pictured with a sexy model on an American flag. That did it, I no longer have any respect for him.

After Donald, Ted Turner became my male ideal. Even though he is a bit of a rebel, I liked him. He does a lot of good things with his money. He goes after what he wants and gets it. Like when he pursued Jane Fonda. Nothing is to unattainable to him. He has donated large sums to charity and more than that, oversees how it is spent. I think every man in this country with that kind of cash should do that. Then he too divorced Jane, the woman he chased after for so long for a bit of fluff. I have no problem with anyone divorcing their mate, but do it for a good reason not because you have "hot pants". How can we look up to these super men when all they use their money for is to get into the pants of some young super model!

I think at the moment my only famous ideal men are Mel Gibson, & Tom Hanks they both seem to have figured out how to handle being a celebrity, good husband and father fairly well. I also like Al Gore, I knew little about him until the last election, but I voted for him and wish he had won. I think he would have made a great president. He has class, brains, scruples, good looks, spirituality and compassion.

I have no use for Bush, who thinks he beat him.

Among my personal friends and acquaintances, both new and old their are several women I admire greatly.

The first is my friend Patty. Like most of the women I've known for a long time, divorce was an absolute No, No to her. We were brought up that way. I have known Patty for about thirty five years, since our oldest son's were in Parochial school together. She was married for over twenty five years, and had five children.

Her husband was a selfish, homely, greedy Italian man. He seldom helped her. He was always scheming to make money. Patty was always cleaning house, her home was always spotless, she worked with me in the P.T.O. and in the school. She was extremely religious, from a very Irish background.

Her parents were very nice a little more wealthy than mine had been, so she did go to college for nursing but most of the time did not work while the kids were little. She was a little younger than I. She kept up her nurses license and helped in the school sometimes as a school nurse.

She had a big house and was always scrubbing and cooking. Her husband liked his food and his wine. Patty put on a lot of little parties and social events for friends and family. Her husband was always starting a project around the house and then leaving it half done forever much to her chagrin. Sometimes if Patty expressed displeasure with him or the house he would buy her a little present but it was something she didn't want or that never fit. I remember her showing me a huge robe he bought her one time. You could have fit three of her in it.

Eventually his constant drinking led to abusive behavior not only toward Patty and the kids but toward neighbors and acquaintances. Patty was upset and surprised when I got my divorce but a few years later she did the same thing. She was devastated by it, even though it was necessary. I think for a while she felt like she had failed at being a wife and mother. No one in her family had ever gotten a divorce. Most of our friends thought the same thing. Once the divorce was final however, she really rallied. She got a great job on the Police force as a matron and nurse, and eventually was put in charge of the rape unit. She is still working it although looking forward to retirement. She put all of her children through college by herself and bought a great little house where she can decorate and garden.

We often travel together and she still entertains our friends at little dinner parties. One of her daughters was in the Peace Corps, while she was stationed in Africa. Pat went over and spent two weeks in a native African village living exactly as the people did.
Sleeping on a straw mat on a hut floor, using a toilet that was just a hole in the ground, and eating what they ate. I'm always telling her not to let her children take advantage of her, because she is so easy going she won't ever tell them no. I love her and look up to her. She does need to take better care of herself.

We also have something else in common we each have a gay son. When she first found out, she called me because she knew my son had been out for a while. She didn't know how to handle it. He wanted to come home and have a wedding. She was afraid her Irish relatives would die. I told her to welcome him home with open arms and don't let anyone say anything. I'm sure it took a lot of courage on her part, but she did it.

Now he and his partner live near her and have adopted an adorable black baby. He is so cute and its a riot to see him dancing the Irish jig. I once told her a gay son, never leaves his mother like your other sons do. He is always there for you.

As her parents got older their sole care rested on Patty's shoulders, despite a great sacrifice to herself she cared for them until they passed away, along with taking care of herself, her job and the kids and grandkids. She somehow manages to do it all. I hope eventually she will have more time for herself and take care of herself. She has also taken care of a sister who has been suffering from a brain tumor for many years. And during another friends bouts with cancer took her for chemo a lot. She never says no, her hands are crippled with arthritis, and she has other health problems, but I have never seen her without a smile on her face. She likes being alone, has no desire to get a man. I think her deep spirituality gets her over her trials. God bless you Pat I love you.

The next person I admire is my friend Phyllis, as different from Pat as night from day, although they have had some similar life experiences ! Phyllis is a tiny little thing, great little figure probably a size two. I have only known her for three or four years. As long as I have been going to the singles clubs. She has become one of my closest friends because we are very much alike. We like the same music, we both love wild, different clothes, we both love to go out, and dance. We both love to eat sweets.

Phyllis has been on her own about fifteen years or more. She had only two children I think both girls. She has her own home and has no desire to ever marry again, but loves to date and have the company of men. We do not like the same type in men, which is good because for sure we would have been competing if we did. She likes big husky men, tall. I like short, dark men. Phyllis is close to my age, and she is the only woman I know who goes out more than I do. She not only goes out three or so times with me, but she goes to the Country western line dances and lots more. It keeps her in fine shape.

She is very attractive and has great long dark full hair. I would give my eye teeth for. My hair is thin and straggly and blonde. Her only problem, as far as appearance is she used to love to sit in the sun and as a result has suffered some sun damage to her skin that she very much regrets. It doesn't stop her from still being attractive. She used to be a hair dresser in her earlier years, now she works retail. She gave up her career to have her children.

Her husband was a very controlling and mentally abusive man (so she said,) she put up with him for many years because she was afraid of him. Eventually she left him, she went to her mothers and never looked back.

She is feisty, determined, and very capable. She and her ex are friendly these days, he helps her out sometimes with her home. She is very social but does not feel the need to have a man around on a permanent basis. I admire her for what she is now. Extremely attractive, fiercely independent, funny, fantastic dresser, very talented, and a loyal friend. She can handle herself in any situation. She has many suitors or admirers that have followed her around for years. We have a lot of fun together. She and Jimmy are good friends and tease the hell out of each other. We love you Phyllis.

Another friend I have sort of lost track of but greatly admire is my friend Vinnie. She had been divorce for some years, at the time I met her. I've now known her for maybe four years. Her husband divorced her at a time when their only son was dying of Aids.

This "wonderful " man ran off with his much younger secretary while his son was dying! No woman would ever do that, but I could relate, because many years before, my husband had an affair when my young son was dying of leukemia! Some if you neglect them for any reason will run to another woman! They don't have the patience or the ethics to wait till the bad situation is over. Most women would not have been able to bare up under that kind of strain, but Vinnie did.

Her son passed away some time ago now. He was her only child. Alone, no child no husband, she got herself a job in a supermarket. She is now a manager and still works there. She is another very tiny little woman like Phyllis. She is very Italian. Very attractive I believe she is in her late 50's but she looks fantastic and dresses impeccably.

Mr. Wonderful, her ex recently took her to court, because he now has a new young wife and a couple of babies and he wanted the court to drop his alimony to Vinnie because he couldn't afford it. Luckily the court found for Vinnie.

When I was first divorced Vinnie was one of the girls who took me out and introduced me to the different singles clubs and dances. During the time we were going there she contacted cancer on her face. They had to cut out a big hunk of her face. Anyone else would have been laid up for months. Not Vinnie, she put a great big bandage over her cheek and dressed all up and went to the dance anyway. I was so proud of her. She is a beautiful and attractive woman and most women would never have had the guts to go out that way, but she did and lots of guys asked her to dance anyway. Because she was still smiling and pleasant. After several setbacks and another operation she finally got rid of it. Today you cannot tell, there are no noticeable scars and she is gorgeous. She has recently met a man she has been dating a while. I have not seen her for a while but I drop into the super market now and again to check on her. She deserves the best, her son did leave her a lovely grandson and wife that give her as much support as they can. She has true beauty and class, keeps herself in great shape and dresses like a million dollars. She is one of my heroes!

My fourth lady that I admire is an old acquaintance, but a new friend. During the time that I was married to my second husband, I naturally became acquainted with his nieces and nephews, some of whom were the same age as my husband. His sister and mother had babies at the same time. This gave me a niece that was four or five years older than me. We had a small family but not necessarily a close one.

This niece, Barbara had grown up with my husband like a sister, but she always called him uncle so I became aunt. During the sixteen years I was married, although I had always thought she was absolutely gorgeous, Barbara and I had not been very close. We were casual friends, we occasionally got together she and her boyfriend of twelve years and my husband and I.

After my divorce I lost track of her for a while, but I heard that she and her boyfriend had broken up. I called, she was depressed and felt her life was over. I encouraged her to come to the singles, but she didn't think she wanted to. She had been married twice and both of her previous husbands had passed away. Now with this third long term relationship gone she just didn't think she had the energy to start over again. She really felt at the time that she was too old to go to the singles.

Jim and I kept at her, one night she finally went. She was an instant success, the guys were all over her, she looked like a movie star. She started dating, but at the beginning she was disappointed that not all the guys were reliable, and honest. After three or four different guys had taken her out, she began to feel that there were no good guys out there. In the meantime however, she was shopping and dressing in a more youthful way. Wearing her skirts a little shorter, and loosing a little weight although she didn't need to. She was very popular, but she was looking for Prince Charming.

Then one week we talked her into going to a new place. Jim even went all the way to her house to pick her up because she didn't want to drive the 50 miles to our house. That night she met him Prince Charming. Ron he was a little doll and they clicked right off the bat. For a short time there was a little concern about the difference in their ages, Ron was only 53 but after dating her for a few months he realized it did not matter, she was as energetic and full of life as he was. They have been going out over a year now, they have taken trips together, met each others families and having a great time. They both love socializing and dancing. It's truly a love match. I admire her because she didn't give up, she was willing to go out on a limb to give life another chance. She didn't close herself off from new experiences. She keeps herself attractive and youthful, helps her children and grandchildren. She is extremely sexy, she is pleasant, understanding and a good friend. She is also very spiritual, she attends church every Sunday as I do. We love you Barbara and Ron, your a great couple, good luck.

Another lady I need to tell you about that I admire greatly and aspire to be like is Eleanor my youngest sister. Eleanor grew up in the same dysfunctional family I did. She was only about nine when my mother ran away. My other sister and I tried to raise her for a while, but when we left to get married, she pretty much had to raise herself and help out her father and younger brother.

She was always a girl with a great attitude and great sense of humor. I had only been married a few years when she came to me one day and told me she was pregnant! She was only sixteen at the time and I knew my step father was going to go nuts and probably kill the boy. The boy was an attractive but poor kid from the wrong side of the tracks, I liked him alot but doubted that my father would. I went to where my step-dad worked and told him. I had to literally hold him down but eventually he got over it and the kids got married.

That's what you did in those days, no baby was ever born out of wedlock. As time went on her husband proved to be a hard worker and good husband and father. They lived a decent life for almost fifteen years. Then her husband lost his job, they lived on the other side of my stepfather's house. When their first son was about nine years old. They had two more babies, a boy and a girl only about nine months apart. After a year or so of unemployment my sister went to work. Her husband could not take having her working and him staying home, even though he was a better housekeeper and better at taking care of the babies than my sister. It just wasn't done in those days.

His brothers and other guy pals started teasing him about being a stay at home dad. He couldn't take it and started drinking and taking dope. The rest of the story I have told you earlier in the book, he was murdered in Colorado.

What I admire is the way she turned her life around after that. Getting a good job with the phone company, looking after three kids by herself, getting over the trauma of the previous years. Then opening her own coffee shop and raising her kids. She became involved with a very nice guy, although early on he was a challenge too. They never married but he was there for her , helping her to raise her children and making a home.

They have been together twenty three years now the kids are gone and they have six grandchildren. They own a nice home where they entertain often. We go to a lot of family get-togethers there. We went there for Thanksgiving this year she had twenty three people. Her kids are great I love them all. Despite the fact that her health is not great, she has sugar diabetes and arthritis, she never gives up. She still works out, plays golf, pool and darts.

She drives a good fifty miles back and forth to work every day, she still works for the phone company. She takes her grandchildren a lot and is constantly buying them something or doing something for them. They socialize a lot with friends, and travel when they can. Last year they played pool in a tournament in Vegas. My sister is extremely generous with charities. Every year she goes and gets a truck full of turkeys for the town welfare program in her home town for Christmas. She has done this for many years. She volunteered her time for shut-ins, she drives an alcoholic who lost his license to and from work everyday so he won't loose his job. Until she got sugar she gave bone marrow on a regular basis. She makes me look like a selfish bitch.

She is also very spiritual, she says the rosary everyday and goes to church on Sunday. She has a great sense of humor and keeps you laughing with her hilarious stories, generally stories making fun of something she did. She has little patience with things that are not right with the world in general, she is a strict disciplinarian with her children and grandchildren. No one takes advantage of her, she doesn't put up with any shit from anyone. She is a short fat little person but would take on a seven foot man if need be. She is constantly trying to improve herself both physically and mentally. She has lost 60 pounds in the past year. I love her dearly and am very proud of her. I hope she will be with me a very long time.

The last two women I have to mention in the women I most admire are my two daughters

They are good examples of today's women, struggling in their own environment for survival. They have more education than we did, but their problems are the same, they are trying to raise children by themselves in a terrible world. The pressures and stresses are different, but just as overwhelming. I see them doing this, and I wish I could relieve them of their burden but I cannot. All I can do, is offer encouragement, advice, and the assurance that this too shall pass.

Both of my daughters have my grit and integrity and survival skills.

They are both great examples to all women.

My oldest daughter Kelly, was educated as a special needs teacher, she married her child hood sweetheart, also a teacher. They started their careers together, in a tiny town in New Hampshire. At first, it was a story book life, they were married for a couple of years and bought a little house and then started their family. My son in law who was a sweet nice boy, I had known since he was sixteen, was always jealous of Kelly's accomplishments. I think was a little happy when she quit working to have a family. The only exception being, he didn't like having all the support depend on him.

Kelly was the perfect wife and mother. They had three children in all, one girl and two boys. By the time the third baby came, her husband was anxious to have her return to work, to help him support them. This is when the disagreements began. During those early years I often warned him quietly that he was going down the wrong path. He had taken it particularly bad when Kelly's father and I divorced but I could see him making all the same mistakes.

During the summers, when her husband was out of school, Kelly had always taken a job as a waitress to help out, but he didn't like baby sitting the kids while she did this. She would come home and find the babies still up at 10:00, dirty dishes in the sink and the house strewn with toys.

Eventually they broke up. He was devastated, but by the time it happened she was fed up. They were probably married about fifteen years. He had been a better father than my husband, but his temper, his lack of patience, his smoking, drinking with his friends, decline in his health and lack of interest in fixing it, weight gain, disinterest in his wife's concerns, not wanting to address the problems eventually caused her to fall out of love with him and to run out of patience with him.

Now she shines, but works her head off, she works two or three jobs, is on the school committee, plays woman's hockey, teaches aerobics, takes her three children to all their activities and manages to juggle a new boy friend. She is beautiful, her children are well adjusted, she is a great daughter, she is tired, and stressed beyond understanding but she continues. I hope she has the strength to see it through to the end. She is a beautiful woman inside and out, she takes great care in her health and appearance, and does a great job with her kids. I am extremely proud of her. She recently appeared in a magazine layout for her physical makeover, she is forty two and looks twenty five, her beau is twenty eight.

My second daughter, Christy, three years younger than Kelly and always in her shadow, or so she thinks, was always the rebel. She was extremely sweet and somewhat fragile as a child. We called her "weinnie", as a child because she was tiny and pale. We always worried about her, and when her older brother got leukemia at six years old, his teacher, who also had Chrissy said she would not have been surprised if I told her Chrissy had it, but Kip looked so healthy!

But Chrissy was strong, and defiant, she married a man I could not stand. I even refused to go to the wedding until the last minute. I was always respectful to him but I knew he was not husband and father material from day one. He was from a wealthy family and was a spoiled brat. Selfish and basically lazy, he would rather go hunting than work. My daughter became a respiratory therapist, which was a major accomplishment for her, because she was not a good student and studying came hard to her. It made me twice as proud when she accomplished her goal.

They bought a house and her husband went to work as a plumber, only because his father owned a plumbing supply store and that was the easiest choice for him. My daughter worked in several hospitals, until she decided to start a family. Once she had her babies, (she had two a boy and a girl a couple of years apart), she worked two twelve hour shifts on the weekend so she could be home with her children during the week.

Her husband often refused to stay with the children on the weekend and would often call her at work, in the emergency room to come home. In those days she often called me or other family members in tears because of his behavior. Eventually they also divorced. He became physically abusive.

She has continued to progress in her career and is doing a wonderful job raising her two children despite his still being a pain. She has been divorced at least ten years. She is engaged to a wonderful man, she bought a condo for her and the children and works long hard hours to support them.

She and I are best friends, I give her a lot of constructive advice. I'm sure she thinks I am overly critical but I hate to see her stress so much. I want her to take it easy and less seriously. She is beautiful, keeps herself in great looking condition, but has a lot of health problems that I worry about. I hope she can hold in there a couple of more years till her children are grown and then she can taste the fruit of her labors. I love her very much and worry about her constantly. I admire her courage, and determination and stamina. I know that their is a lot of sibling rivalry between she and her sister but there is not need for it. They are both doing fantastic jobs and each has their strengths and weaknesses and they should be each others biggest fans.

Well, I think I have given you a good example of the type of women I admire. None of these women are people who have set the world on fire doing some heroic work, like mother Theresa or someone, but I think that's the point. We each in our own way, can be a hero to someone, we can each make the world a better place if we just take care of our little parcel to the best of our ability and try to do our mundane jobs with humor and example.

Whatever cross, God gives you to bare, do it with class, humility, and pride.

This is the example I am trying to impart, make your little corner of the world better and the whole world will be. A positive attitude, a change for the better.

Now of course there are people who will not change! They are right even if everyone else in the world has a different opinion and even if you can show them they are wrong. They would prefer to sit in their misery and become more miserable. Everything is someone else's fault, not there's. They are insecure, afraid, stubborn, and lazy. They have no confidence, they are afraid to stick their head out of the sand. Its too late for them, they are "happy" with the way things are. It's none of our business, everyone can't be like us! You don't know what you are talking about! You can offer to help, you can talk till your blue in the face. They will not budge. They use every excuse in the book.

I do not admire these people. If you try your best and fail at least you tried. Not to try, I have no respect for. The names have been changed to protect the innocent. Maybe I am being judgmental, maybe there are extenuating circumstances I do not know about but most of these women I have known for between four and thirty years. In the five years I have been going to the singles I have met a few hundred women, many of whom also have these traits. They are not attractive, they are not productive and they keep these ladies from leading a full, well-rounded life. We all need friends; we all need to do things outside of our daily routines or we will grow fat, lazy, tired and unhappy. So really think about these types I am going to tell you about, and if you see yourself in them, try to get rid of it.

The first thing is negativity. Two of my very best friends in the world are very negative people. For years when I am having a conversation with them, if we have a difference of opinion, I give them my opinion and if they continue to argue the point I eventually give in and let them have it because I know unless I can show it to them right there in black and white they will never accept my opinion on the subject.

One of the things that I learned when I was in politics was to do my homework when I had an opinion about something. I am a very opinionated person but I found if I wanted to have other people accept my opinion I had to verify it. These people I am talking about do not do that. They just have an opinion and that is that. You accept it. Not only are they opinionated but they are negative. Nothing is ever going to work, nothing is ever correct, especially their husbands or ex-husbands. Their husbands don't know anything but neither do their friends. They are always right, you are wrong.

They know everything about everything and everybody. They wonder why they don't have any friends left after a while or why when they call someone to do something with them they are always busy. These ladies may be extremely bright and very knowledgeable but not usually very happy or content. If they have a problem, you can give advice but they will never take it unless they thought of it first.

When you're having drinks or lunch with a friend there should be give and take. If they give you an opinion, at least consider it. If they say you should go this way and you think that way, don't insist on going your way. Find out the correct way. If your friend says, "You look good in that," say, "Really?" and get a second opinion. Don't say, "Oh no, I would never wear that." Give and take, that's the way it should be. Maybe that is why you got divorced in the first place!

The second type I want to tell you about is the bitter, depressed and most of all vengeful woman. She can never close the door and get on with her life, even if she was the one who wanted the divorce. I have met many women like this at the singles and also among personal friends. When their marriage started to go downhill, they didn't know what to do about it. In some cases, maybe they decided it was a mistake to get married in the first place. Maybe they came from such a dysfunctional family themselves they had no skills to keep their marriage together. At any rate, eventually the woman walks out, leaving the children with the husband. She does this for many reasons. Maybe the husband did not want the divorce and wouldn't leave. Maybe she knew she could not work and take care of the kids. Maybe the kids wouldn't go. Maybe it was financial. Maybe she just was sick of it.

At any rate, she leaves, but forever after wants revenge. She still blames the husband for the break-up and spends the rest of her life finding ways to make his life miserable. You can never get on with your life as long as you hold grudges. You can never get on with your life as long as half of your life is still taken up with "how to get back at him." This type of woman does not want to see her ex with another woman, or her children. She wants him to continue to pay for everything for both her and the children. She will take him back to court at the drop of a hat if she can. You will seldom see her out with another man, because every man she meets has to listen to her bitter divorce story and how awful her ex is. When a man meets a new woman, he wants her to be stress-free and fun, not bitter and vengeful.

It is also never a good idea for either a man or a woman to talk about the other spouse in a bad way to the children. Children are not stupid. They know if Daddy is an asshole or not. They know if he is good to them. They know if he has a girlfriend, and they know if he says bad things about Mummy. Eventually, no matter how young they are, they will figure it out. I know this from personal experience, my own and that of many friends. It may take a few years but the kids eventually figure out for themselves who is the better parent or if you are both good or bad parents. But the one who for years has been saying untrue or bad things about the other one will eventually be discovered by the children, and then it could come back on you, so don't ever do that. On the other hand, if Daddy is an asshole and you try to say nice things about him, eventually the day will come when the kids will tell you, "Daddy is an asshole." So remember revenge destroys; it wastes your life. We only get one life. It goes by way too quickly. Make the most of it. Don't waste it on unproductive and negative things. Forgiveness takes a lot, but it feels good and it's productive.

Don't be greedy. If you meet a man and he can't afford to take you to the best places, let him pick the place. Let him know that he can plan things that don't cost money. If you make more than him, be willing to pay once in a while. Now I am not talking about a guy who has plenty of money and is a cheap s.o.b. We never tolerate that!! I'm talking about a nice guy who may be recently divorced and is trying to balance child support with his new singles life and is dying to get to know you but can't afford a $100.00 dinner every week. Be helpful to him in managing his dates and money. I meet so many girls at the singles who just walk up to a guy and say "Buy me a drink.". If he asks them out, the girls tell him where they want to go and it's usually some real expensive place that they can't afford themselves so they get a guy to take them. A week later they are back complaining that the guy never called them again. I wonder why.

Then there are the whiners. Do you know any of them? I never met one until I started going to the singles. With all the women I knew when my children were growing up, I never met a whiner.

We were all young mothers, bringing our children up in middle class neighborhoods. In our crowd we were all Catholic, our children all went to parochial school. We all worked in the PTO raising money for the school with activities. We were the Brownie moms, the Cub Scout moms, etc. We all had big families and we all worked hard.

The whiners were a new breed. Maybe they were wealthy when they were married and had maids and nannies, I don't know. All I know is they can't do anything for themselves now. Every time you meet them they tell you all their miseries. They never feel good. They go to the fortune teller to find out what's in store for them tomorrow. They are always late and always look like an unmade bed, yet they pay astronomical money for everything. They make all kinds of promises but can just never get to it. They are dying to meet men, but they bore the men with the same whiney complaints and the guys take off. They are always asking you to fix them up. They are bold enough. They will walk up to a guy, but they don't know how to carry on a conversation without telling them all their troubles. God forbid they ever have a real catastrophe because they could never handle it. They want to please but don't know how to go about it. They are not particularly nice to service people like waitresses, bartenders, or salespeople. It's like they expect them to be there to serve them. If you are a whiner, stop right now and listen to yourself. Think of something interesting to say that is not a complaint or problem. Smile, be cheerful, and put out that damn cigarette.

Some people I want to cover that I do not admire are people who stay married who shouldn't. Now you may think that sounds kind of contradictory since that should be everyone's goal when we marry—to stay married. But while some people get divorced who shouldn't, there are people who should not stay married.

I know personally several people who are living in abusive marriages. A couple of the girls I have known many many years. When I first knew them they were happy, cheerful women looking forward to being married, raising children and having the American dream. For a few the American dream turned into an American nightmare, and after many years in an abusive relationship, these ladies have lost so much of their self-esteem they may never get out from under.

One, and I know there are many more than her, is in a sexually, physically and mentally abusive marriage. She has stayed in it because she does not want the community or her friends or family to know.

She pretends that everything is all right and she buys herself expensive gifts to make herself feel better, but it never works. After so many years she thinks it's okay because they are getting beyond the age where sex is a part of their daily lives. But he hasn't changed and he has grandchildren, and I wonder what will happen if she dies before him and the kids still bring the grandchildren over.

We have a responsibility to do something about abusive people.

Another girl I know is physically abused by her husband weekly. He smacks her around. She has had so many injuries she can barely walk. She dresses beautifully, she fixes herself up and smiles prettily, but she is always on the verge of tears. All I have to say is, "How are you doing?" and she breaks down. I have given her information on shelters and all sorts of other ideas, but like the other girl she is afraid that she will have no place to go or that he will follow her. You must understand the courts are fair. In an abusive relationship they are more than fair. Half of everything you have with your husband, stocks, property, homes, cars, pensions, is yours. The court will give it to you. You do not have to depend on him to give it to you.

You do not have to get an attorney or make a big fuss. Go to the family court, get the paperwork, make it out and return it. Get copies of everything that shows what you own. Go to a shelter if you think that is necessary. If you are not afraid of your husband, get a place, move your stuff in and start the process. No person should have to live in an abusive relationship, no matter what. There are women who are in mentally abusive relationships. This is a little harder to understand or put into words, but it is just as destructive. Maybe your husband is a drunk or takes drugs or loves verbally abusing you or putting you down all the time, or picking on the children or animals. I have known men who killed their wives' pets just to upset them. Or they are verbally or physically abusive to the children. There are all sorts of abuse, but you do not have to put up with any of it. I remember one time when a Catholic friend of mine said to me, "Mary So and So is a saint. She has lived with that drunken, abusive man for twenty-five years!" I said, "I'm sorry, Mary is not a saint. Mary is an idiot." She was shocked and didn't like my remark. That was the mindset that people grew up with in my day. You stayed with your husband no matter what. He could be cutting off your fingers one a day. You were faithful; you stayed with him. You never complained, you worked your ass off, you had twelve children and when you were finally, completely worn out, no good to anyone either mentally or physically, he divorced you for another woman.

Thank God we've come a long way, baby. We are no longer in the dark ages. If you see yourself in any of these scenarios, please take stock and do something about it.

Chapter eighteen:

The power of a woman!

What's lost today, may be won tomorrow, Miguel de Cervantes(1547-1616) Spanish writer

    Women have unlimited power over men. Ever since Eve, you may think so now, but really think about it. If you can't really relate, you need to work on it. Your power is untapped. You must have had it as a young woman, you can get it back. Or if your a late bloomer like me and you really never were aware of it, we must cultivate it, because it is a fact.
    Think over the ages, how many men have been brought to power or to devastation by a woman? They always say, behind every successful man is a woman. That is true, but it is also true wars have been fought over women. Kingdoms have fallen over women. It's not the woman's fault, its the choices men make! But we sure can influence those choices.
    Adam and Eve, Sampson and Delilah, Antony and Cleopatra, Romeo and Juliet, The Duke and Duchess of Windsor, Charles and Camilla, Kennedy and Marilyn, and of course Bill and Monica. The list goes on and on, how can you doubt your power. Men gave up everything for these women, kingdoms, money, power even their souls.
    Gary Hart ruined his chances for the presidency, Jim Baker lost his power, money, following and wound up in Jail. Bill Clinton could have gone down in history as one of the greatest presidents but instead he will always be remembered for his indiscretions. Donald Trump might have run if he hadn't been doing sleazy things with a model,

Even my hero Rudolph Guilliani governor of New York, was running against Hilary and then it came out he was having an affair and a really nasty story followed. The power we have, and the common sense not to behave the way men do. Men cannot resist us ladies, that gives you unlimited power. You may not be feeling that power right now, but you can get it back, it doesn't matter if your twenty or eighty you just need to believe in yourself. Make yourself look as good as you can, exercise, diet, eat right, dress right, work on your self esteem, confidence, sense of humor. You'll feel it come surging back, The Power!! When you are using your power over men, however be sure they are respecting you. No one respects, Monica. She's made a lot of money but she will always be a joke. Remember the more they cannot have it the more they want it. Use your powers for good not evil.

It's only when we truly know and understand that we have a limited time on earth-----and that we have no way of knowing when our time is up---that we will begin to live each day to the fullest, as if it was the only one we had, Elizabeth Kuhler-ross (1926) Swiss born, American psychiatrist

Chapter nineteen:

Depression:

Sometimes, no matter how hard we try we still get depressed. Our lives are very stressful now a days. Older women like ourselves who have not been in the work force for long, may have many real things to worry about. How will I retire, how will I support myself, I have no Health Ins. My car is on the fritz, I need an operation I have arthritis, a bad back, allergies etc. It can't be helped and its ok to allow for a little depression.

Give yourself a day, baby yourself. Feel sorry for yourself, call your best girlfriend and cry on her shoulder. Try not to do it on your boyfriend but if you have to! He will not understand the way a girl friend would. Maybe these things have no solutions, the thing is you can't solve them by worrying.

If you cannot do anything about them, let them be and when the problem comes deal with it instead of worrying before. You have no health ins. you have looked into it in every way and you cannot get it. Getting stressed over it ahead of time, will not help. It might even make you sick, then where are you. Keep yourself as healthy as you can. Take vitamins, get plenty of rest, and lots of vegetables, fruits and water. If you get sick and have to go to the hospital they will have to give you charity.

You can't afford an apartment, car, groceries apply for aid and if you don't get it move in with a friend, relative or one of the kids. Your lonely go out put on your best smile, make some new friends. The point, everyone gets depressed, your not alone, don't make a habit of it. Unless you have a chemical or physical reason you can overcome it. If you can't shake it go to the doctor, find out if you are bipolar or have some other reason for it. Last resort take medication.

As I get older and go to anniversary parties, and high school reunions etc. I keep coming across old friends or class mates or acquaintances that I haven't seen in as many as maybe twenty years. When they see me, they cannot get over how good I look or how much energy I have or how happy I appear to be. They tell me all their health problems, and other problems and then they tell me how lucky I am. I tell them, it's not luck its attitude, it's work, its having a reason to get up every day. It's believing your still 20 or 30. You don't get thinner or in better shape because of luck you get that way because you work at it.

These people, many of them, don't go out of the house except to go out to eat! They do not exercise their minds or bodies and then they wonder why they don't feel well. Think young, listen to music, talk to people who talk about something other than their grandchildren and their aches and pains.

Don't keep putting it off till tomorrow. Start today in what ever capacity you are able. Here's a good suggestion and it won't cost as much as you think. Jim and I took a cruise this year to the Mediterranean. We started in Lisbon Portugal, went to Barcelona, Spain, Gibraltar, Morocco, the French and Spanish Riviera's and wound up in Italy. The entire trip for two weeks was about $3,000.00 but I'm not recommending it for the places it went but for the atmosphere that was on the ship. Mostly older couples, but they did a lot of traveling and they were so youth oriented. They did a lot of walking, dancing, talking, played games, we put on a show. Everyone on that ship had a great time and did everything including people over eighty years old and people in wheel chairs.

We were at a party recently when my fiancée commented to me. They are a very emotional family aren't they? They cry at the least little thing. I told him yes, but when they had a chance to face up to their problems and do something about it they wouldn't. I have a close girlfriend who has emphysema, her dad died of it. She is a heavy smoker. She told me when her dad died she vowed she would never get that disease, it had been so hard on her watching him. She did not give up her smoking however and now she has it. I keep at her all the time to give up the cigarettes, so far she won't but I'm praying. She complains of her skin tone, and texture and blames it on hormones. But it's not hormones it's cigarettes and sun worshipping. If you don't smoke you will not have tiny wrinkles and dry dead looking skin, the cigarettes take all the moisture out of your skin. It cuts off the blood supply to your skin. I realize this is a very hard habit to break but today their are all sorts of aids to help so please stop.

When young people die of lung cancer, their family is there at the wake crying why us, we have such bad luck. It's not luck it's choice choose wisely. It doesn't help in the dating scene either, I have another girl friend who is a heavy smoker, neither Phyllis or I have ever smoked. This girl will be sitting with us and trying to meet a guy, puffing away non stop on the cigarettes. More than one guy has told me and Phyllis after we introduced her to them. I won't date a girl who smokes. Then she cries to us, why can't I get a man, you guys are so lucky!! Give me a break!! Take care of the problems before they happen, and maybe you will have "Good luck" too.

If it becomes necessary to sell a big house, because of a death or divorce , maybe one of your adult children is living there, or the house is full of "stuff" that you don't want to part with. You need to do what is right for yourself and your financial situation for the rest of your life. I know its hard to part with "stuff" that's been around for many years, but look at it like a new adventure.

I have several friends who have paid money to "store" their "stuff" for up to ten years. They don't even know what is there anymore. When you move into a new smaller house or condo. Tell yourself you are going to have everything new if you can afford it and give away or sell all the old stuff. It will make you feel better. Memories are not necessarily good and the ones that are, you can fill one box and take with you.

Let your adult child fend for himself, If you have "stuff" that you would like to remain in the family what better time than now to give it away. I even cleaned out all my old pictures, I made an album for each of my grandchildren, with pictures of all of their old relatives on both sides so they will know where they came from. I put some of their baby pictures, pictures of their parents and aunts and uncles when they were little. They absolutely loved it. It saved me a lot of storage and I will know that the kids will have those memories.

If I had died, God knows what would have eventually happened to all those old pictures. Get rid of everything else you don't need in your smaller place, don't save it "in case", you will never again own a big house! Get something you can manage and afford for yourself. Don't listen to children who try to make you feel guilty. "How can you sell that?" We grew up there, we love that house! Our memories are there! That part of your life is gone, start your new life with new "stuff". Dream up a great looking "Bachelorette Pad", you should see mine. My living room is purple, with red fringed lampshades, my bedroom looks like an Indian sultans room. Make your surroundings happy, comfortable and stress free. Remember we make our own luck and solve our own depression.

Chapter twenty:

Men they can't all be bad!

When I hear somebody sigh: "Life is hard", I am always tempted to ask, "Compared to what?" Sydney Harris (1917) Newspaper columnist

My last chapter I am dedicating to men. Probably none of them will read this book, but I don't want to leave out half the population. Men are wonderful and fascinating creatures. Sometimes they get a bad rap. The problem is we measure them by women's standards.

You can't they are not capable of behaving like a woman. My life if full of them, and at different times and different stages of life they can be wonderful or awful! Little boys are sweet and loving, especially to their mothers. They are fun and inquisitive and they would just as soon bake or do dishes as play ball or play with trucks. So are old men, when men get old they return to their little boy behavior and are just as sweet.

In between old and young is where they give you the problems. because that is when they are strutting their manhood, and behaving like the wild stallions they think they are. They like to think that they are all unique and different and in someways they are, if your talking about looks. If you are talking about behavior, they are all the same, as if cut from one mold. That's why so many comedians tell jokes about them, they all leave the toilet seat up and never clean the bathroom, they all put the toilet paper roll on backwards, they all refuse to ask directions, They are all exhibitionists, especially where their privates are concerned. They can't help it they were born that way. Most of them do the best they can with their limited abilities, and what we teach them. Most men can't stand listening to a woman talk for more than a couple of minutes no matter how interesting she is. All the time she is talking they are looking at her but they are not listening. Its a well know fact that women use their much smaller brains to a higher capacity than a man uses his larger one. Women use many more words in a day, They express themselves better they listen better.

We must remember by nature men are hunters, explorers and fertilizers. Without their sperm we cannot reproduce. Men are fun, frustrating and loveable. Some try much harder than others. In recent years with women going out into the work place more, more men are becoming stay at home dads or at least helping out. It's good for them and good for the kids. The children get to know their dad's better and have a better relationship.

With the discovery of such good information from sources like" Men are from Mars, women are from Venus", we are trying to understand the opposite sex a little better. They are trying, some of them to understand us to be more patient and to help with the child rearing. We want them to be more sensitive then we comment on it when he is or think he's not strong if he's sensitive. Don't expect him to do it like you do it, let him do it his way, be patient and compliment him on it. A lot of times they don't help because we won't let them or we look like we have it in control. Try saying, "will you help me with this"? If he doesn't then get on him. They'll offer to do the dishes or clear the table and we'll say, "Oh no that's ok I have it". More than once and they won't offer anymore, I know that's what happened to me.

I took a great helpful man and turned him into a couch potato. They offer to bathe the baby hand him over. The more we say, "No I'll get it" the less they will offer. I know most women do that all the time. Then they complain that they are overworked. Compliment them for everything they do for you even if you think you could do it better. Men it's easy to please a woman, it really is. Listen to her, or pretend to listen. You don't have to comment, just agree, give her sympathy if it's a problem. Occasionally surprise her with one flower or a card for no reason. Leave a card on the seat of her car to find in the morning when she goes out.

What points that will give you! Or bring one home from work. If you hear her say we are out of something, like milk or anything, bring it home without her asking. Be fair about television shows, don't always hog the remote. Go to a women's movie once in a while, especially if she's been to the last five action films with you. We think they are so senseless. The main one that will get you so many points, compliment, compliment, compliment. Nothing goes further than a sincere sounding compliment. You look gorgeous tonight, the meal was wonderful, the house looks nice, goes a long way. I have met many wonderful men in my lifetime.

I have also met a lot of jerks. The jerks don't last in my life very long, because they get told off in spades in a hurry. I have three wonderful sons, I tried to bring them up to be aware of a woman's feelings most of them help out at home and are pretty sensitive and caring. Two of them love to cook and do most of their cooking at their respective homes. I think compared to the men in their fathers generation they are considerate of their partners and do more than their father did. There is always room for improvement and you know if your good or not. My boys are terrific I am proud of all of them.

Then there is Jim my one and only, he is one in a million. He is very tuned into my feelings, he listens and helps out around the house. He can cook, iron, clean, and do dishes better than I can. But, I am very guilty of not letting him do things and I think I am making him lazy. I make his lunch every night, which he will happily make if I don't. I generally do the cleaning and ironing so its never there for him to do. I do have to nag him to take out the trash and clean his bathroom, but I think when we were first together. I was always telling him, "No I'll do it". I try to stop doing that as often.

He jumps in to make the bed in the morning, he does anything he can to make my life better. He scratches my back, and massages me. He is handsome, he takes good care of himself. He dresses like a million dollars, and he always thinks of spontaneous fun things to do. He takes me out dancing two or three times a week, to the movies, out to dinner at least once a week. He leaves me little notes in my lunch bag, my car, the mail box. He doesn't take me for granted. I try to do the same thing for him, because only if you both try all the time will things stay exciting and new.

We both talk and flirt innocently with other people, to keep us sharp and in the groove. It's fun. He is friendly to my family and friends and me to his. My kids love him. He fits in anywhere. I don't complain about his golf or card playing and he in turn lets me go off with my friends, if he doesn't want to do what ever it is.

He isn't the only good guy out there, I know at least half a dozen, and they are always telling me they are looking for a good woman. You just have to meet them half way, don't start a relationship with a chip on your shoulder because of the last guy. If I had given up after my last divorce, because I thought I was too old or too fat or too anything I would never have found all the great guys I did and especially Jimmy.

One of my friends has been stressing over the fact that a much younger man has been chasing after her for the past month or so. He is gorgeous, smart, talented, everything you would want in a guy. He is twenty five years younger than she is. She keeps turning him down because he is too young. I told her go for it. You don't have to marry the guy, enjoy his attention, have a good time, fall in love, have great sex, see where it goes. Men have been doing it for years. Women find it difficult, when we go out with a younger guy all we see if our kids.

But as women age better and continue to have great energy into their sixties and seventies we are going to have to pick younger men. In all the time I have been dating I have only found one man may age that has the energy I have. My friend Tony, he can keep up with all of us old broads and the younger ones. But me, Phyllis, Barb and most of our friends are dating men five to fifteen years younger. My cut off age is forty, I won't go out with anyone younger than my child.

So seize the moment. Go out with anyone you are attracted to try to keep age out of it. See where it goes. Have dinner, go to a show, how many more chances will you get in this lifetime? So go for the gusto while you can!

It's been four years since I started on this book. During that time I have put into effect personally everything I have told you. Not only in my own life but with many of my friends. Many of them have had major life changes. Not totally through my intervention but with our advice and through our example, or just dragging them kicking and screaming through what they needed.

My sixty seven year old niece after a two year courtship has recently moved in with her fifty four year old gorgeous boy friend. She had been a recluse, sitting behind closed doors thinking her life was over when her spouse of twelve years left her. We literally went and got her and dragged her to a club. She became popular, dropped about ten pounds, and started dressing much more youthful. She dated a few men and then without warning Mr. Right appeared.

My younger sister was at a point when I thought she would be a cripple. She had lost interest in herself and looked twenty years older than she was. At fifty two she was living in elderly housing with her disabled husband. I took her in, got her a job where I worked. She began to take an interest in herself, her sense of humor returned, she took some courses, got a job. Today she and her husband are living in their own trailer very happily. She is still working.

A very close friend was in dire straights, she had lost her job unfairly. I got her a job, she sued the place that fired her and won. Today she is still working at the new place and got a settlement large enough to put her on her way. My ex has settled down in Miami with a wealthy woman five years his senior he met at the club, who is exactly what he was looking for. My girl friend Vin is celebrating three years with a great guy she met at the club.

More and more of our friends are settling down in new lives with new people and new situations to the point that Phyllis and I now sit on our stools every Friday and Saturday night saying where has everybody gone!

Most of the ones we still see, are looking for that evasive Mr. or Mrs. Perfect, or they are afraid to take a chance again. They got hurt once and won't step up to the plate. They are afraid of settling down and losing their freedom. Settling down or being monogamous does not have to mean losing your freedom. Set up the rules at the beginning. Unless the person you have picked is very possessive, (and if they are run like hell in the other direction), you can enjoy the love and companionship of another person without giving up any of the freedom you enjoyed being single.

Make up your mind what you want to do with the rest of your life, and express that to your suitors. You'll find one that shares your desires. Remember though that you have to return the favor. You have to allow them to enjoy what they like also.

You can have as much, or as little freedom as you want but you have to tell them that right up front. Jimmy knew the first date we had that I intend to travel and go dancing three nights a week forever. I knew the first date that he had a great love for golf, and I had better let him play! We are going on four years in our co-habitation and we still get along great. He goes off for a week or two to play golf every year with the guys. He also plays a couple of times a week. I go dancing, he comes with me one or two nights but when I want to go more often than that, I go alone.

We never ask each other, who did you dance with, who's that girl you are talking to etc. We tell each other everything we did when we were absent from each other, we introduce one another to new friends of either sex that we meet. I am gracious to other women he knows, he is gracious to other men I know. We both know that the other one is not being unfaithful. At our age if it ever got to that we would just go our own way with someone new.

We are not married, we each have our own money, we share the bills. If your boyfriend likes to drink, gamble watch sports, don't think he is going to give these things up because he starts going out with you. He might by your example but not by your nagging. Chances are these things may have had something to do with his wife leaving him in the first place. You have to be the woman he wants that lets him have his passions and he has to respect yours. Start talking about these things the minute you meet. Your old enough to know now that people do not change, not a lot anyway.

Everyone is not interested in a man, and the girls I know who are not, have settled into good jobs, have made peace with their lifestyles are doing what they want and are happy with themselves. We have a great network of girlfriends who travel together, get together for parties or go out to dinner. These women, like my friends Pat and Peggy have become very successful in the business world and are supporting themselves very well through their own hard work and determination. One was married twenty five years and had five children, the other thirty seven years and had nine children.

Jim and I are celebrating four year together, we met at a singles club. I wear his engagement ring as a symbol of my dedication of being monogamous with him. We don't intend to marry, but who knows. The important thing is I have found the one man in the world who compliments me and understands me. He is always there for me both physically and mentally yet he doesn't put restrictions on me. I can do anything I want without him hassling me and in return I don't hassle him.

We have in the past four years traveled to Austria, and Bavaria, China, France, Africa, Italy, and Spain together. But he has also taken his golf trips with the guys and I have gone off to Vegas with the girls. I tried to take up golf, but I am terrible at it. I do enjoy the exercise so when it's a couples tournament I will go with him. It will never be the passion with me that it is with him. But, I tried.

He goes dancing with me, but when he's tired of it I go alone. We both do our best to get along with each other's children. This is necessary, because between us we have nine.

We both love movies so we go at least once a week to the latest flick. We both still go to the singles club together and "hold court" at our favorite stools. All night long people come up to us and talk or ask advice. We are always surrounded by single friends or ex's who's company we still enjoy so we go there. We find the most prevalent mistake people make is being too judgmental too soon. They judge all the new people they meet by what has happened to them in the past.

You cannot do that. This new person you just met had nothing to do with what caused your divorce or why the guy you met last week didn't call. They may also be completely innocent of why they got divorced. Do not listen to what anyone else tells you about someone new you meet. Get to know them with a completely open mind. Make your own judgments only after you have gotten to know them.

If another woman there was rejected by a guy, and then he shows interest in you, the first thing she is going to do, is come over and tell you, "He's and asshole", and proceed to tell you why. Jealousy is a terrible thing. Men do the same thing. Just this past week I took a very attractive friend of mine to the singles for the first time. I introduced her around. Immediately she was a hit with the guys, they surrounded her like "dogs in heat". When she chose to dance with one of them, the others came up to me and said. What's she dancing with him for? He's an asshole, I told them all, if he is she will find out.

She didn't need them to tell her that. She's a big girl, she's been around, and even if she hadn't she would learn. I have had many girls come up to me when I was with a particular guy, before Jimmy. He's a drinker, he's a liar, a bum, he's cheap etc. I thank them but proceed to find out for myself. Sometimes they are right, but more often than not the guy didn't like them so they have to get back at him for rejecting them.

I would have lost out on some great friendships if I believed what everybody told me. Most women still make the mistake of hassling a guy who takes their number and then doesn't call them. Or making promises they don't keep. Take this all in stride and don't let it throw you. Take the attitude when a guy takes your number that he won't call, don't seem too eager. It's a game guys play at the singles, how many phone numbers can you get in a night. Sometimes by the time they get home they've lost them, or they go into the laundry on a napkin the next day. I've know guys who spent weeks looking for a number they put in the laundry. If you don't expect it it will happen.

You only want the good ones to call, If you see them at singles the next week don't even mention it. If they want to call they will come up and tell you they lost it, otherwise ignore the whole thing.

I have made a pretty good name for myself in my job. I went from the collection agency where I started, to a medical billing place, to a hospital and now I am a Chiropractic assistant. All self taught. Each time I changed jobs I looked for something a little better than the last. I tried to learn with each job. I did not take something that was well outside my reach. I was never afraid to go out at age 64 now and try to get something new. I always get the job with the interview. My last two jobs at the hospital and for the doctor I won at the interview. Both times their were as many as twenty other girls, younger, more qualified, more experienced. But I relaxed, let my sense of humor, and confidence show through. Fake confidence if you have to work on it, put your mind in a calm state. Tell them your strengths, older people can generally point to a good work ethic that a lot of young people don't have. They don't have to worry about you moving on, or getting pregnant. I have a perfect attendance work record. Stress these things, if you live nearby tell them. If you have no ties like a husband and children pulling on you that's all a plus. You will be surprised at how well you can pull it off.

I have a good relationship going with most of my children and grandchildren. My oldest granddaughter is seventeen! Both of my granddaughters come to grandma to borrow clothes for parties. They like my clothes much better than their mothers. All of the kids have had problems most of them have been divorced themselves. I try not to give too much advice, but I cannot always hold my tongue. If I've been there and done that I tell them. They can take my advice or not. I don't get my feelings hurt, if I feel it's necessary to tell them something I do. I am still their mother. They have to make their own mistakes however and in the end they will. I don't let it influence my life too much and I would never let them move in.

I am always trying new and exciting things, I would love to write a column for a newspaper, or travel and give seminars to women's groups. I would love to go to Law school, but I'm too lazy. The important thing is keep happy, keep fit, keep active. The latest thing on people living to be over one hundred is they kept active.

I just read an article on another woman's idea of how an over forty year old woman should dress, I got a kick out of it so I will share it with you.

She said, animal prints, short skirts, and blonde hair are not appropriate for business. B.S. I'm here to tell you, I wear all of the above and more so. It's all about image, and the image you want to portray. I know that animal prints, short skirts and blonde hair are not typically accepted business images. That is the image, I want to portray, and I am a good business woman in spite of that. I find people have fun with it. A woman or a man who maybe would not wear that themselves still get a kick out of seeing someone else wearing it. I wear novelty jeans and wild tops and big jewelry to work all the time. My patients expect it and when I don't even the most conservative ones express disappointment. They love to see what I am wearing today. I prefer a sexy or bohemian image at my age to a typical business suit. It is not me. It will never be me, and I don't care what some feminist thinks. You can be the image you want to be, and show them you are brilliant even if you look like Marilyn Monroe. Look at Erin Brockovitch. These are the "you" years, the fun years when you don't have to answer to anyone. You may have to live with a "dress code" in your office but within that dress code there are many options. And when you're not in the office go nuts.

At the moment I am looking forward to new challenges, traveling around the world. I want to meet as many new and exciting people as I can. Before I die I want to go as many places and have as many new experiences as possible. Don't let the world situation clip your wings. Me and Jimmy went to China two weeks after 9-11 and had no problems at all. I hope someday to partially retire, but if I can't no big loss. I hope before I die to contribute something to the world that they will remember me by. If I can't I am at least confident that a lot of people will remember me in some small way.